A WORK OF ART

A WORK OF ART

Art Herriford

iUniverse, Inc.

New York Lincoln Shanghai

A WORK OF ART

Copyright © 2005 by Art Herriford

iUniverse books may be ordered through booksellers or by contacting:

iUniverse
2021 Pine Lake Road, Suite 100
Lincoln, NE 68512
www.iuniverse.com
1-800-Authors (1-800-288-4677)

ISBN: 0-595-34242-6

Printed in the United States of America

Contents

FOREWORD

It's been a lifelong thought process of mine to put my thoughts down on paper about the life I've led. It's been many years in the making…83 to be exact.

Call this my "Artobiography" if you will.

It amazes me that so many changes have taken place over my lifetime…my schooling, my navy experiences, my family, friends…and I wanted to share those with everyone who has been and is a part of my life to make this book possible. There are so many to thank, so many to remember, I just can't name them all. But they know who they are, and how much gratitude I have for them being in my life.

I hope these pages bring you some joy, some memories, and some insight about the type of person I am.

It was not only a "work of art…" but also a labor of love to have written this.

Art

1

The Beginning

In Cleveland, Oklahoma on the morning of 17 April 1922, at 4:15 AM, Arthur Gerald Herriford and Edna Naomi (Kendall) Herriford were blessed with the arrival of their first-born child: A son who would bear the name of his father. To begin with, I was rather sickly during the early days of my life. I am not sure of the cause early on, but according to my mother, it nearly took my life.

Art Sr. stood about six feet tall and weighed approximately 200 pounds. Soon after I was born, he developed rheumatism and was in such pain, that when his dad sent him to Claremore, Oklahoma to take the mineral baths, he was transported to the train on a stretcher. Upon returning from Claremore some 30 days later he was walking upright. To my knowledge, he was never again bothered with rheumatism although, in later years he developed a heart condition related to rheumatic fever. Dad was born in Indian Territory, (Oklahoma) on 18 October 1900.

My Dad was the eldest of five children. Next to him was Lyle, then his only sister, Marguerite followed by Maurice and finally Alvis Booth (Al). Al is younger than myself by 2 months, 3 weeks, and 2 days. I lived much of my life, off and on up through mid-teens with my father's parents. Dad worked the oil fields, and was therefore away from home for long periods during the various oil booms. He would move Mother and us children in with his parents and be gone.

My mother was born in Little Rock, Arkansas on January 21, 1903. She stood 4 feet ten and a half inches tall, and let me tell you she never failed to emphasize that half inch. She was well liked by everyone who knew her, always with a smile on her face and a very outgoing personality. Mother carried the nickname "Midge", but also answered to "Oma". Everyone in Cleveland, a town of twenty-five hundred souls knew her. You see, my mother worked as a waitress in the leading cafe in town, seven nights a week, 12 hours a night for one dollar a night. She did not however, start slinging hash until I was about ten years old.

There were four of us children. I being the eldest was followed by sister, Dorothy Jean, born 8 October 1925. Next was Richard Roy, born in January 1930, followed by Patty Jo, born 12 July 1933. Dick was killed in a hunting accident in November 1945 at age 15. He was my paternal grandfather's buddy. Granddad Herriford took his death very hard. After a period of time, he took my youngest sister, Patty Jo under his wing, and they became very close.

Mother came from a large family consisting of three girls and six boys. To the best of my knowledge, their order of birth follows: Joe, Mother (Naomi), Ted, Clara Belle, Dudley, Lenny, Dorman, Berbie, and Elmer Page. I do not know when Dudley passed away. I visited him and his family in San Diego in the summer of 1946 and never saw him again after that. Joe predeceased Mother by about five years and she passed away on 31 March 1980.

Some of my first recollections were that we lived on the second floor, above an oilfield Tool and Supply Company, on the main street of Cleveland. My grandparent's house was located two blocks west on "B" avenue. Cleveland in those days looked like a forest of oil derricks. For most part the derricks were constructed of wood, about 85 feet high. Later on steel pipe was utilized to construct the derricks. There was between four and eight oil wells within each city block. Cleveland was known as "The Pioneer Oil City of Oklahoma", and perhaps still is referred to as such. It could have become the "Oil Capital of the World" as Tulsa has become known, had not the city fathers opposed development and wished to keep it a bedroom community.

In the early 1930's all the oil derricks within the city were torn down. Actually this effort was spread over a period of five years. Power houses were built at various locations with rod lines running over the surface of the ground. Pump jacks for 10 to 18 wells were thus simultaneously powered by a single source to pump oil. Some of these wells were located 4 or 5 blocks away from the power house.

Granddad Herriford was in the grocery and feed store business about the time I was born. Dad worked for him as butcher and clerk. While Granddad was good at purchasing, Dad's forte was selling. Together they made a good team until Dad started working the oil fields. Nearly everyone bought on credit and paid their grocery and feed bills at the end of each month. The stock market crash in October 1929 put Granddad out of business. Years later I came across an old trunk in the loft of the barn loaded with old credit records for grocery and feed bills totaling in excess of thirty thousand dollars. By current standards, that was a very large sum of money. Additionally the local savings and loan went bankrupt, taking another sixty-five thousand dollars in the process.

I recall Dad had an old dog, a Bloodhound named Prince. Dad used to take Prince up town with him, go to the post office, obtain the mail and give it to Prince to take home. One story was told, that on his way home one day, other dogs accosted Prince who put the mail down, placed one front paw on it and pivoted around keeping an eye on the other dogs, never removing his paw from the mail. Finally, the other dogs moved on after which Prince picked up the mail and continued on home.

2

West Texas

You have heard the term "Spare the rod and spoil the child". Well the rod was never spared on either side of my family. Let me say, none of us children was ever abused in any way, but if we stepped out of line, you can bet our bottoms got warmed. Once when my mother was going to give my brother, Dick, a switching, Granddad Herriford volunteered to get the switch from a peach tree out back of the house. When Mother started applying the switch to Dick's backside the switch started breaking off in about six inch lengths. It seems that Granddad had been carried away with this project and his pocketknife had partially cut through the wood at various lengths along the length of the switch. Both he and Mother could not keep from laughing and thus ended Dick's punishment.

Once during my first year of high school, (9ᵗʰ Grade) Dad found out I had been cutting class. He took me to the principal and told him if he saw fit to whip my butt, you could bet I would get another when I got home.

At this point, I would like to make a statement to the effect that I believe a great injustice has been foisted upon our children with the elimination of corporal punishment in our school system. There was discipline in our schools before. Today the schools have lost all control over the students. Since abolishment of corporal punishment, the achievement of students in our public school system have sunken to an all time low. Think about it.

Early on, we kids were assigned chores. Some must be performed prior to going to school in the morning, while the bulk required time after school. As for myself, besides milking the cow or two we kept in town from the farm, both morning and evening, stalls must be cleaned out and new straw bedding put down. The animals must be fed and sometimes included a new calf that had to be weaned from nursing and taught to feed and drink on his own. We cooked and heated the house with wood stoves. Therefore, it was necessary to carry enough wood for both stoves into the house to last through the following day. For most part the wood had to be cut and split before it could be taken into the house. My Uncle Al and I usually shared this chore. During the summer months, it fell my lot to plant and tend the garden as an added chore. Gardening was my project for my class in "Future Farmers of America" (FFA) early on in high school. In order to get into this class one had to know "When does a pullet become a hen?" The answer is, when she loses her first foot race.

In 1926, my dad went to Pampa, Texas, which was in the throws of a big oil boom. He sent for my mother, sister Dorothy one year old and me, age four to come out and live in the Texas panhandle. Dad had left a 1923 "T" model Ford coupe in Cleveland when he went west, so my uncle Maurice proceeded to drive us to Pampa. In those days there were no paved roads. A first class highway was gravel surface. The bulk of all roads were graded dirt and sometimes nothing but a trail across the prairie. The distance was approximately 300 miles to Pampa. It was the fall season and there had been lots of rain. The roads were often times full of ruts and in low places, muddy water completely covered the roadway. Several times, we became stuck and a farmer would pull us out with his team of horses. I recall on one occasion a farmer used his Fordson tractor. Nearly every time we paid one or two dollars for this service. The first night we spent in Fairview, Oklahoma having driven about ten hours during the day. I recall that it was cold and had rained a day or two before. The route we took was US-64 to Enid, Oklahoma then US-60 from there to Pampa, Texas. The total trip distance was 292 miles. We arrived in Pampa late the second day where we were met by my dad.

Dad had contracted with a carpenter and his wife to build us a "boxcar" house in a small settlement of oil field workers on the lease where he worked. Dimensions of the single room house were approximately 30 by 15 feet, set on blocks about 2 feet off the ground. A curtain was strung across the mid-part of the single room in order to separate the bedroom area from the kitchen and living spaces. For about two weeks, we lived in a boarding house on the south edge of Pampa while the house was being completed. Our new house was located about 8 miles south of Pampa. There was no inside plumbing, except for natural gas that had been piped from a caseinghead gasoline plant down under the hill to the south. This provided fuel for cooking, heating, and lighting. Mantels mounted on a ceramic base and packaged in a little round cardboard container, purchased at the grocery store were necessary for mounting on gas fixtures to provide lights.

It was necessary for Dad to guy the house down such that it would not blow away during the violent wind storms we experienced from time to time. A water line had been run along with the gas line into the settlement and a few spickets capable of being drained had been installed in packing boxes to prevent freezing, were our source of water. However, on several occasions during the winter the lines still froze necessitating people to go to a pumping well with an ax and cut holes through about a foot of ice in the circulating tank for the well engine cooling system, to get potable water. These were redwood tanks with a capacity of about a thousand barrels. Let me tell you that when it gets cold in West Texas, it is <u>damned</u> cold. There was nothing to stop the wind but the barbed wire fences and they were all down.

I mentioned earlier there was no inside plumbing. Back of our house about a hundred yards was a canyon, the depth of which was about 60 to 70 feet, having a width of between 100 and 150 yards. The banks were eroded back about ten to fifteen yards before the sides became vertical for perhaps 40 to 50 feet. Considerable sagebrush and mesquite afforded privacy. This then became our toilet. Actually, it was the privy for the entire settlement although it required coordination amongst all of us. Our biggest concern during the summer months was rattlesnakes, of which there were plenty.

Across the canyon was located another settlement of six or eight dwellings. I recall on one occasion a man over there was drunk and having words with his wife. We could hear them shouting across the canyon. The man got into his car and was backing it down the slope toward the lip of the canyon, trying to get it started. Everyone on both sides was afraid he was going over the side and were yelling for all they were worth. He got the car started a short distance from the edge however, and took off.

On another occasion, our immediate neighbor parked his 1925 model Chevrolet coupe with disk wheels next to his house when he came home from work. Apparently, he did not set the emergency brake nor did he leave it in gear. Below us, about 150 yards were several families living in tents spread over wood frames who were in the process of building more permanent dwellings. One had dug a hole in the ground preparatory to building a cellar. I was playing near our stoop when all at once I detected Mr. Rainwater's car begin to back down the slope. I started yelling, but it was too late, his car backed into the cellar excavation. Next day a tractor brought from some place on the lease towed it out. By the way, my dad hung the initials "I.P." on Mr. Rainwater and that became his nickname all over the lease.

Sometime after my 5th birthday, 17 April 1927 the Rainwater's were making plans to leave the area. Their house was up for sale, and the constable in Pampa being interested, came out to look the place over. I was out playing between our houses when he arrived and introduced himself to Mrs. Rainwater. my mother called me into the house and asked me if I knew what he was doing there. Having overheard his introduction, it has been told I remarked that he was over there "constipating around". For sometime thereafter I was said to be the source of that quotation around the neighborhood.

I recall Dad coming home from work and jacking up one rear wheel of the car. This was to make it easier to crank next morning. Also during the winter months, a teakettle of boiling water was taken out and poured over the intake manifold so the engine would start more readily. Cranking a "T" model Ford in those days was tricky business. Many men wound up with broken arms as a result of engine backfire causing the crank to kick backward striking the arm.

3

1926 Pampa Oil Boom

Early in the spring of 1926, we took a trip to Lipscomb, Texas to visit my Great Uncle Roy and Aunt Ella Branson. They lived on a large cattle ranch. To the best of my knowledge, we stayed about a week. It was quite an experience watching the cowhands work the cattle, which on one occasion were being fed cotton seed cake. I recall an incident Aunt Ella told about Uncle Roy that had her scared out of her wits. They purchased and had just received shipment of nine Brahma bulls and Uncle Roy had put them all in a common corral next to the barn. Unfortunately, the bulls began to fight among themselves, so in order to protect their investment Uncle Roy grabbed a pitchfork and climbed into the corral. Single handedly he managed to separate the bulls and got two each in separate corrals and one in the barn, after which they settled down.

The trip to Lipscomb was quite memorable in several respects. In the first place, the road leading out of Pampa after a few miles turned from a graded surface to a wagon track across the prairie. No doubt you have seen in movies, a post with names painted on small boards pointing in the direction of various towns? Well this was common in those days. The distance to the various settlements however, was seldom ever displayed and maps were rare. We left home about daybreak and arrived at the ranch between nine and ten p.m. that evening. The total distance approximated 100 miles. On one occasion, I recall a long snake stretched across both wheel tracks of the road. The front wheels of the car hit it, but it was gone before the rear wheels got to where it was. Another time just after dark had settled in, Dad brought the car to a stop and cautioned Mother and us kids to be very quite. There was a large herd of long horn cattle drifting across the wagon trail. Dad was too scared to shut the car engine off for fear of spooking them into a stampede. I do not remember how long we sat there, but it was a very long time. Finally, we arrived in Lipscomb needing gasoline. There was but a single filling station in town and the owner did not want to get out of bed to sell us fuel. With some haggling and the promise of an extra dollar or two, the fellow came out and started cranking his pump. Dad paid him and we proceeded to the ranch, about 15 miles further.

Dad traded the 1923 Ford coupe for a new Ford roadster in the fall of 1927. Shortly thereafter he received word his mother was quite ill. He threw some things into the car and headed for Oklahoma, leaving Mother and us kids at home. He was gone about 6 days. On the way home, the trunk cover on the roadster came off and Dad just kept driving. He did not stop to pick it up, but rather had it replaced when he returned to Pampa. One day we were on our way into Pampa to do the weekly grocery shopping, etc, Dad's paycheck blew out of his shirt pocket out across the prairie. Dad did not even bother to retrieve it, the wind being what it was. He had enough cash to cover our shopping needs. The next day he had the company cancel the lost check and issue a replacement.

Another time Mother and a neighbor lady drove 6 or 8 miles to a farm to purchase buttermilk. They had heard good things about this farmer's dairy products, and we all liked buttermilk. However, upon leaving the farm, the two women having bought a gallon of buttermilk each, after driving some distance from the farm stopped the car and poured out their purchases after noticing the buttermilk was loaded with flies.

I recall the only way to transport crude oil to the refineries in those days was by rail. Unlike today, pipelines only covered very short distances. One late afternoon when we were in Pampa, a train of oil cars was experiencing great difficulty getting through town. The locomotive was a Double-Mally, or what we called a double engine. I was told a hog had been hit and dragged along the tracks for some distance lubricating the rails thus causing the locomotive drive wheels to lose traction. Each time the engineer tried to apply power the drive wheels would spin with no traction.

After coming to a stop what was left of the hog was removed from the cowcatcher, the rails were cleaned and sanded and the train then slowly moved out of town. This and various things I have mentioned above are recollections of a 5 year old boy in the wild and wooly town of Pampa, Texas during the oil boom of 1926 and 1927. Pampa at this time was a typical wild west cow town, with boardwalks, hitch rails, and false fronted buildings. The main street, two blocks long was not even graded nor was there a jail. Law enforcement took over the livery stable and converted it to a makeshift jail during the early part of the oil boom. Posts were set either side of a stall with a sucker rod between. Inmates were shackled to the rod and slept on hay laid down in the stalls. Dad's job ended in the fall of 1927 and we moved back to Cleveland, Oklahoma.

Following that, Dad and my Uncle Maurice obtained work in Kansas City, Missouri. We traveled by train to get there. About this time, Mother cut down and sewed me a suit from one of Dad's old ones. I remember how proud I was wearing my new suit. One Sunday we were riding the street car out to the zoo when a little black girl sat down in the seat beside me. I was quite startled. Mother said later that the expression on my face was something to behold. Our apartment building contained several black families. Being from a state south of the

Mason-Dixon Line this was all new to me. Soon however, I got used to it although I cannot say I accepted it at the time. Over the years, I must say that I have been privileged to work and socialize with people of all races and ethnic backgrounds whom I greatly admire and respect. Unfortunately, I still cannot condone interracial marriages between blacks and whites.

When I was about six years old, mother and dad would let me visit my maternal grandparents for two and three weeks at a time during the summer months. They lived about fifteen miles southwest of Cleveland on an oil lease where Granddad Kendall was the Pumper. He had 12 or 15 wells that were his responsibility to keep pumping around the clock. There was no proration in those days, which later allowed wells to pump a restricted number of hours a day in order to preserve the oil field and keep from pumping it dry.

My uncle Ted had a model "T" Ford that he would drive to Cleveland every week or so for groceries and other provisions. My folks every once in a while would let me go back home with him. He was living with my grandparents at the time. my mother's younger brother, Elmer was about two years older than me and we got along fine with one another and had fun times playing there in the country. We used to obtain barrel hoops and fashion a "T" bar handle of laths with which we would roll those hoops all over the place. For lack of toys in those days, we managed to fashion our own.

The various wells on the lease had their own peculiar sounds when pumping. On several occasions, I recall during the night one of them would shut down. Instantly my grandfather would wake up from a sound sleep and remark to Grandmother or anyone else for that matter, the identity of the well that had shut down. The wells pumped day and night in those days, except when one would be shut down for pulling rods and tubing permitting repair of the pump located in the bottom of the well. Granddad would get up, dress and go to work to bring the well back on line.

Grandmother washed clothes by hand and heated water in an old cast iron pot over a fire in the back yard. It was incumbent upon us kids to carry water in pails from a large storage tank about 75 yards from the house. On one trip I stumbled and fell against a jagged pipe protruding from a packing box at the base of the tank. I was wearing short pants and the result was a gash about 4 inches long just above the knee on the outside of my right leg.

4

Growing Up

Dad's youngest brother, Alvis Booth known as A.B. during our growing up years, were for the most part raised together. We are more like
brothers than uncle and nephew. The result of all this is that all his and
Millie's kids call me Uncle Art. Several of them were grown and married before they knew I am a cousin rather than an uncle.

Anyway, Al and I along with Aunt Ella and Uncle Roy Branson's
two youngest boys, Mike and Glen, (Pat) were all four about the same
age. Al was 2 months, 3 weeks and 2 days younger than me. Mike was
somewhere in between and Pat was about 18 months younger than
myself. The four of us boys enjoyed growing up together although we
were not continuously in contact with one another. Ella and Roy were
my Great Aunt and Uncle who lived on the farm about three miles
south of town, town being Cleveland, Oklahoma. They moved onto
the farm that was handed down on my dad's maternal side of the family. All this was after they were forced off the ranch in West Texas by
the great depression. Years later, in the spring of 1940 to be more precise, another son of Aunt Ella and Uncle Roy, Jack who was about 6
years older than I, we each enlisted in the US Navy about 6 weeks apart
unbeknownst to one another. Jack went through boot camp at Great
Lakes, (Chicago) and I at San Diego, Naval Training Centers. More
later on this subject.

When I was about 12 years old an incident occurred that really
caught my interest. Two brothers from Cleveland had enlisted in the

Navy and were somewhere in California when one was struck and killed by a car. The other brother escorted the body back home and fulfilled the duties of "Military Honor Guard" at the funeral. I attended the funeral and was very impressed by the deportment of the surviving brother. From that moment on I was convinced that if I ever should enter military service it would be the Navy.

We boys worked on the farms at various times during the summer and on weekends chopping weeds in cotton or cornfields and cutting fire wood to get us through the winter. There were three other farms aside from that where Aunt Ella and Uncle Roy lived. They belonged to the paternal side of my dad's family. One belonged to my granddad, one to his brother, Charlie and one to their sister, Emma. Uncle Charlie lived on and farmed his own place until his death while the other two places were leased out to share croppers, except for the 60 acre hay meadow on granddad's farm. I helped put up hay during the summer months and helped Uncle Roy pick corn in the fall. I have a scar on my left little finger caused by a corn husking tool. After Uncle Charlie's death, Uncle Roy farmed his place along with the farm they lived on.

While there was little money to be had in those days, generally speaking we had a healthy life. Never did any of us go hungry unless we were away from home looking for work, etc. We raised plenty of garden produce, had our own beef and hogs that we butchered, in addition to raising our own chickens. One must keep in mind that while we usually ate well there was a terrible lot of work necessary to produce our food.

The depression of '29 that dragged on until the early 1940's was a very harsh experience for everyone, except perhaps for the very wealthy. Many times, I had put cardboard in my shoes to cover holes in the soles, so I could go to school. Twice I took over my dad's shoes that he left at home when he was away working in the oil fields. To say the least, he was not very happy with my wearing his expensive shoes.

About age 14, I obtained a morning paper route for the Tulsa World having about 40 customers. It was necessary for me to get up at 3:00a.m. and go to the Quality Cafe where the papers were dropped off from the delivery truck. After devoting 30 minutes to folding papers, I would set out on foot to cover my 3-mile route carrying two paper bags, one on each side. Normally I would finish in time to return home for breakfast then go to school. I collected on Saturday morning, 35 cents a week for each customer for which I paid 25 cents for the paper. Assuming 40 customers, I netted $4.00 a week, providing everyone paid me, which they seldom did.

I had one customer, a plain nasty old man who would call me every kind of foul name he could think of if his paper was not on his front porch by 5:45 each morning. Several times, I tried to drop him as a customer, but my Paper Manager would not hear of it. On rainy days I had to crawl on hands and knees to get up a slick muddy bank having an incline approximating 30 degrees about 30 feet long. Otherwise, I could walk an additional half mile to get through, just to deliver that old man's paper.

5

The Teen Years

My mother was working nights as a waitress at the Quality Cafe, 12 hours a night, and seven nights a week for one dollar a night Some friction had developed at the grandparents and my dad was away working an oil boom. I do not remember just where. In any case, Mother decided it was time for us to move out on our own. Dad was seldom home and there was little or no money being sent. At this point, I believe she had made up her mind to divorce. I had turned 15 and in all those years my dad, except for approximately 3 years had dumped us on his parents every time the going got a little rough. Then he would take off for some job away from home for several months at a time. Although he sent money from time to time, it usually was not much. My paternal grandparents were great people to put up with us. However, they had been too good to their children when they were growing up. They should have booted their kids out and made them look after their own responsibilities rather than bring them home to mother and dad. Still those were some wonderful years in most respects.

Mother found a little house furnished and with money Dad had sent we moved.

R.B. Ott lived next door to us. He was an only child approximately 1 year older than I was. His folks owned a 1930 model "A" Ford, which he drove most of the time. He and I commenced buddying around together. We collected scrap iron and sold it to a junk yard to make gasoline money. In early June of 1937, his folks took both R.B.and me out to his mother's parents farm near Billings, Oklahoma about 75 miles northwest of Cleveland.

They raised wheat and R.B. was slated to work with them through the harvest. They could not however hire me, so I had his folks drop me off in town as they started their return trip home. Within 30 minutes, an elderly woman hired me to work the harvest on her and her husband's 320-acre farm. The pay was $2.50 per day and board & room. That was 50 cents a day more than R.B. was being paid.

After 67 years, I cannot remember the name of the people I worked for. They were both into their seventies and very active. Unless you are a part of it all, it is impossible for a person to realize the amount of work that is accomplished each and every day during harvest season. In the first place, when wheat or oats mature to the point of being ready to harvest, and for that matter the month prior to, the farmer becomes a nervous wreck with worry. Until the grain is out of the field many things can happen totally destroying a crop. Examples being wind, rain, and fire. Wind and rain can break the stalks thus laying the grain on the ground where it cannot be picked up in the cutting process and as for the latter, lightening or some absent-minded driver traveling along the highway tosses a lighted cigarette from a car, and fields around can go up like a powder keg.

I was first put to work driving a lead tractor in the process of towing a combine out of a marshy spot where it had buried down to it's belly in the mud. Having never driven a tractor before, I immediately parted a 15 foot log chain when the clutch grabbed. It fell to my lot to drive the lead tractor the rest of the day. Normally we cut wheat from about 20 minutes after sun-up, giving the sun time enough to dry the dew so the wheat would thresh, until almost dark when the dew impeded threshing.

Since I was the youngest in the crew, it fell my lot to do the chores both morning and evening. My day began about 3:30a.m. when the Mrs. wakened me. After dressing I would bring 14 head of milk cows and a span of mules out of the pasture into the barn, feed and harness the mules, milk the cows, feed approximately 500 chickens, take the milk to the house where I strained and then put it through the cream separator. Following that, I took the balance of the milk back to the barn where it was fed to a half dozen calves and ten or twelve hogs. Then I returned to the house for breakfast.

Following breakfast, I returned to the barn area where I would load a couple grease guns and a 5 gallon bucket of grease on one of the tractors, drive it to the field, hitch the tractor to the combine, grease all combine fittings, then get to relax for twenty minutes giving the sun time to get high enough above the horizon to dry the dew before we started cutting.

We were fed five meals a day. Breakfast, dinner, and supper were taken at the house and at mid-morning and mid-afternoon, the womenfolk brought lunches to the field, thus giving us a twenty minute break twice a day. Normally we cut grain until almost dark when the dew got the grain so damp it impeded threshing. Following all this, it was my job to again do all the chores I had done in the early morning hours, after which I bathed in the pond, changed into clean clothes, went to the house for dinner; then immediately thereafter, about 10:00 p.m. fell into bed. The foregoing describes the eighteen-hour day I worked to earn $2.50 for my efforts. The money I earned bought my school clothes that fall.

The following summer, 1938, I worked for an outfit on the outskirts of St. John, Kansas, although the pay was not nearly so good, but the hours were not nearly so long either.

Dad returned home and He and Mother divorced. We kids were moved back to the grandparents and mother went to Tulsa to work. When school started that fall, Dad took both Dick and I to Oklahoma City. Dorothy and Patty Jo were left with the grandparents in Cleveland. Dad was living with Ida Rowlett in the second level of a garage apartment she owned. One side of the double garage on the ground level had been converted to living quarters where Dick and I slept. Ida was a grand person. I had the utmost respect for her. She was very good to us two boys.

That fall I started school at Capitol Hill High as a sophomore. I was enjoying the greatest year of my life and had a thirst for knowledge like I never dreamed possible. It was my good fortune to have been selected to sing Bass in the a cappella choir, The Glee Club, the all male chorus, a 16 voice mixed chorus, the male quartet, Bass Solo, and the Vocal Director's church choir at the Second Presbyterian Church of Oklahoma City.

Dad was the "Pro" at the Southwest Park Golf Course. I had no idea he was a golfer until then. Although he was not a touring Pro, he was very good and proceeded to teach me the game. The course was only nine holes, but very popular. I was outfitted with a partial set of clubs Dad had come by, and since I did not have to worry about green fees, balls, etc it was incumbent upon me to play at least nine holes on school days and on weekends 36 holes was not out of the question, weather permitting. Surprisingly I was beginning to shoot in the upper seventies before winter set in, but that was primarily because Dad made it a point to play in my foursome frequently and was always the instructor. Wow! He was a taskmaster, but I learned and his teachings have stuck with me all these years.

During the winter of 1939 the owner of the golf course, Joe Rowlett, former banker and former husband of Ida Rowlett, without notice to anyone sold out. With no forewarning Dad found himself without a job. The depression was still upon us. Work was scarce and many family men were without jobs. It appeared I would have to quit school. For a young kid to earn a living and at the same time go to high school was out of the question in those days.

Having dropped out of school, Dad suggested I enlist in the Army Air Corps. After some thought however, I told him I wanted an education and it seemed to me it took lots of knowledge to build warships and also a lot of know-how to operate them. Getting an education was foremost in my mind. Therefore, my choice was to enlist in the Navy. Dad agreed and the following day he accompanied me to the Navy recruiting office.

I was only 17 years old at that time, and the Navy had just recently raised the minimum age to 18. We tried to fib about my age, and after all the necessary papers were signed, the recruiter informed us the following day that he had sent out to the State Capitol and obtained my birth certificate. He further stated he would keep my application on file and give me a call soon as I turned 18. This left me with about three months to get my things in order.

6

The Navy Calls

My brother, Dick returned to my paternal grandparents in Cleveland where my two sisters were living and I went to Tulsa where my mother was living. I worked a few odd jobs during the next few weeks, and then in March as my birthday was growing close, I went to Cleveland for a couple weeks visit with my grandparents. After that, Dick and I returned to Mother's in Tulsa.

In September 1939, when Great Britain declared war on Hitler, I had the feeling it was only a matter of time until the U.S. would be involved. Furthermore, I was at the age most susceptible of having to fight this war. Neither of these matters escaped my consideration. I was of the opinion that, "them who get there first get the best seats". For that reason and reasons previously stated, I was looking forward to being called by the Navy. Sure enough on Monday morning, 15 April 1940 a Navy Recruiter in Tulsa knocked on the door, and informed me I was to be in Oklahoma City the following morning to take my physical. Mother cried. She said she was planning a birthday party on the 17th, my 18th birthday. Years later she confided in me that she was aware I would never again return home to live. She was so very right.

That afternoon I hitchhiked to Cleveland to see my dad and Grandparents. Dad gave me 50 cents pocket money and bought me a ticket to Oklahoma City (something like $1.25 in those days) on the 5:00a.m. passenger train the following morning. The train arrived in Oklahoma City about 7:30a.m. and I presented myself at the recruiting office at

9:00AM sharp. I passed all the physical requirements, except the minimum weight of 120 pounds. The scales showed me being a couple pounds light. The recruiter told me to go to lunch and eat all the heavy food I could hold and come back at 1:00 pm. I went out and bought a quart of milk and all the bananas my 50-cent piece could purchase. At One O'clock, I managed to tip the scales at 120 pounds, most likely with the aid of the recruiter to some extent.

I was given a TR, (Transportation Request) and boarded a train bound for Dallas, Texas at 4:00 p.m. Upon arriving in Dallas about 10:00 p.m. on the night of 16 April 1940, I was beginning to feel rather hungry. After some time I located an all night restaurant near the recruiting office and settled in there. About 1:00 AM, I apprised the night cook of my purpose in Dallas and the fact that I was broke and hungry. I offered to wash dishes and do some cleaning for something to eat. He would not hear of it, but fixed me up with a good breakfast on the house.

At 9:00 AM, I reported to the recruiting office and again received another physical exam, but this time by a medical doctor. Following that, I was told to go to lunch and return at 1:00 PM. Having no lunch money, it was out of the question for me. There were 25 of us being examined for enlistment in this group and I was the only one not from Texas. Back in the recruiting office about 1:30 p.m., we were given a last chance to back out. None did. The oath of allegiance was administered and I was now in the United States Navy.

Following this, about 3:00 p.m. we were taken to a restaurant for our first meal on the Navy. All we could eat and boy did I tie on the feedbag. After lunch, we were on our own until 9:00 p.m. at which time we were to board a train bound for San Diego, California.

Mind you, this was Wednesday, 17th of April 1940, my 18th birthday. I buddied up with an individual several years older than myself and we spent the remainder of the afternoon and early evening in a bar named "The Covered Wagon", a few blocks from the train station. He loaned me a couple dollars that I would repay on our first payday. There was a barmaid that sat in our booth from time to time who told me, "You sound like a damned Blue Bellied Yankee". Being from Oklahoma, I have never forgotten that remark. We boarded our private pullman car a little before 9:00 PM, after which, it was coupled to a passenger train and shortly thereafter, we were on our way.

We met Thomas and Mrs. Dewey on the trip west. Their private car was coupled to our train in Belen, NM and they were with us until Williams, AZ. He was campaigning for the GOP nomination to run for president at that time. They were taking a short, much needed vacation to the Grand Canyon. Both came into our Pullman car and visited for about twenty minutes.

About 4:00 p.m. on 19 April 1940, our train started down the grade at Cajon Pass about 20 miles northwest of San Bernardino, California. I was treated to one of the most spectacular views it has been my pleasure to observe. There was no smog in those days and the eastern end of the San Gabriel Mountains across the pass was something to behold. The majesty of that scene was breathtaking in its beauty.

Our Pullman car was put on a siding in San Diego before 6:00a.m. on Saturday, 20 April 1940. Promptly at 6:00 AM, several petty officers arrived to transport us by bus to the Detention Unit at the Naval Training Station to begin our Boot Training. First, we were ushered into a barracks to deposit our luggage, then placed in formation and marched to the mess hall where, our first breakfast consisted of baked beans and corn bread. Little did I realize at the moment, that I would in a very short time, look forward to baked beans and corn bread for breakfast on both Wednesday and Saturday mornings.

The twenty-five of us in the initial contingent became the nucleus for formation of the largest training company ever to be put through the San Diego Naval Training Center. It consisted of three platoons of 62 men each for a total of 186 men. Three Chief Petty Officers were assigned as platoon commanders, one of which was the company commander.

Normally the detention period was three weeks. However, for company 40-26 detention stretched to five weeks. During this period we were kept inside a 12-foot high chain link fence where no visitors were permitted.

Initially before being brought into the detention area, new arrivals were taken to the barber shop for their first hair cut, (all of it off), then to clothing issue for initial outfitting of uniforms, and finally to the ships store where you signed a chit for $14.00 worth of toilet articles, etc. That left you with $7.00 out of your first month's pay of $21.00. After returning the 2 dollars to the individual that loaned me that amount in Dallas, I had $5.00 in my pocket. I was one among the first 25 people to arrive for Company 40-26, and it took two weeks to receive enough men to form up the company, therefore for all to receive a minimum of three weeks detention, we initial 25 were kept behind that fence for 5 weeks.

We were drilled in military marching formations from 0615, (6:15 AM) until 1700, (5:00 PM) normally, with breaks at various times to go to the Sick Bay for inoculations or to the dentist or into the barracks for a session of stenciling and rolling clothing and learning to pack a sea bag. House cleaning of the barracks generally was accomplished during a thirty minute period following breakfast. Each individual was assigned certain chores. All personal items had to be kept in your sea bag or ditty bag. Lights were out at 2100, (9:00 PM) with reveille at 0600, (6:00 AM). We were allowed 15 minutes following reveille to accomplish our personal amenities before formation on the grinder for thirty minutes of calisthenics before being marched to the mess hall for breakfast. It was not uncommon, should there be some sort of discrepancy in some facet of our training or the condition of the barracks, for the company commander or one of his assistants to get us out on the grinder for an extra hour of drill at nine or ten o'clock at night.

We twenty-five in the first group to arrive were the first to be taught many of the drudgerous tasks, such as stenciling, rolling, and tying clothing articles for stowing in a sea bag. Also, there was the requirement once a week, usually on Saturday morning, to lay out in a prescribed manner, all items of clothing for personnel inspection. We therefore became instructors for all the subsequent arrivals. This went on for three weeks while the company was being formed. The result of all this experience is that to this day I can pack almost twice the amount of clothing into a given piece of luggage as the average individual.

I was one of the smaller individuals in the company, and as such, following inoculations was constantly kidded that I would crap out on the grinder during drill and have to be carried off. That never happened, and I assisted in that chore on various occasions involving people much larger than I.

Ditty bags were secured to the head of two tiered bunks by the draw lanyards using a single square knot. If, upon inspection, more than one square knot was found to exist in the ditty bag lanyard, demerits were given. It happened that one of the Texans in the original contingent I reported in with was from time to time adding square knots to my Ditty bag lanyard. I learned of this one night at the movies when he was sitting directly behind me talking to one of his buddies. When the movie was over, I dashed out a side door, ran to the far end of the barracks and entered the door nearest to my bunk. Standing in the shadows, I observed this fellow start his mischief. With that, I swung around into the isle of my bunk and as he stood up I planted my right fist to the left side of his head, laying the top of his ear open. He started to raise his fists toward me, but he looked at me in a rather dazed manner, then dropped his arms, turned and walked away. Never again did anyone give me any trouble. This individual outweighed me by about thirty pounds and was an inch or two taller.

We completed our five weeks detention period and became eligible for liberty on weekends in San Diego. Two of my friends wanted tattoos, but on our first liberty, I got them back to the base without such. However, the following weekend they went ashore without me and each was tattooed. Both told me, before the week was out, they wish I had been with them to prevent their exuberance. After a career of nearly twenty-one years in the Navy, I have yet to get my first tattoo. I cannot understand people wanting to mar their skin with such crap.

Upon completion of boot training, people in Company 40-26 were granted ten days leave, providing they could afford it. I could not, and therefore was given orders to the light cruiser USS Detroit, CL-8. The location of Detroit was a mystery. I was taken by motor whaleboat from the Training Station out into San Diego bay and put aboard the destroyer USS Anderson, DD-411 for transportation.

My sea duty had begun. Paul Otto Burch, (I only knew him as Burch until much later in our Naval careers) also of company 40-26 at the Naval Training Center, San Diego was also ordered to the Detroit. While I did not know Burch in boot camp, we became close friends later on and we both became Fire Controlmen. WW-II caused us to go separate ways to other ships and stations, but we were again shipmates, as classmates in the Advanced Fire Control School in Washington, D.C. and again when we were stationed aboard the USS Norton Sound, AVM-1 at Port Hueneme, California. Both of us became Chief Warrant Fire Control Gunners. Both of us retired from the Naval Service on 1 December 1960 with credit for 21 years service. Paul became administrator of his mother's hospital in La Mesa, CA and died at his desk of cardiac arrest 6 months after retiring.

7

First Sea Duty

Burch, myself, and several others from company 40-26 were transported by boat from the Naval Training Station out to the destroyer USS Anderson, DD-411, which was moored in San Diego Bay. We were aboard not more than a couple hours when the ship got under way and put to sea. Neither Burch nor I had any idea where we were going. Finally, it was revealed to us that we were steaming to Pearl Harbor, but it was the following day before this became common knowledge.

As passengers, we were assigned to the amidship deck division and given assignments on the under way watch list. My watch station was Starboard Bridge Lookout, where it was necessary to report to the Officer Of The Deck the sighting of any vessel and from sunset until sunrise, every half hour that the "Starboard Running Light and Mast Head Light are bright lights Sir". Birch, on the other hand, was assigned watches in the Battle Lookout about 40 feet up on the foremast. Both he and someone else standing watches up there heaved their guts out all inside the steel enclosure the first night out, and don't you know the only way in and out of the place was a trap door through the bottom. Anyway the next morning the division Boatswain Mate ordered me to climb the mast and clean up the mess. Well I got as far as sticking my head up through the hatch in the bottom of the Lookout and observed puke about 2 inches deep all over the deck so, back down the mast I went. I told the Boatswain Mate he could have me put in the brig if he so desired, but that I was not about to clean up such a mess made by someone else. He did not object and assigned someone else to the task. To this point I was not bothered by sea sickness but had he insisted I go back up the mast it is my belief that I would have become quite sick.

I was utterly enchanted with the ocean. While I had heard many times about deep blue sea, never until now could I have believed it was so very blue and indeed so very deep in appearance. We encountered both schools of tuna and bottle nosed porpoise. The porpoise swam back and forth across our bow and I'll swear they were scratching themselves on the stem of the ship each time they crossed. The tuna stayed with us for a little while and it was a sight to see so many of them jump clear of the water. They must have been 3 to 5 feet in length. With the activity taking place aboard ship, I still remember a strong sense of serenity associated with the ocean.

Later that first day at sea we rendezvoused with the aircraft carrier USS Enterprise and her escort destroyers. We took up a position on the carrier's starboard beam and remained there most of the afternoon while she launched and recovered aircraft during flight operations. She was quite an impressive ship and in those days her aircraft were all propeller types. Late that afternoon, we left the formation along with the USS Hammond, DD-412 and resumed our course to Pearl Harbor. All at once it dawned upon me that I loved the sea and to this point had not experienced any symptoms of sickness.

There was a ship's cook aboard; Anderson, who was bothered with sea sickness when first putting to sea, had developed a method of overcoming it. He would fix himself three fried egg sandwiches and go aft on the lee side of the ship where a settee was secured to the after deck house. After eating the first sandwich, he would sit until he felt it coming back up, then step over to the rail and heave it up. Returning to the settee he would eat the second sandwich and repeat the process. The third sandwich as a rule stayed down after which, he would be all right the remainder of the trip at sea.

The second morning at sea was pretty rough. The sea had become quite rough during the night, and in keeping with an old destroyer sailor's remarks, our bow was going over one and under two, (waves). The ship would shudder from stem to stern and the roll was something to behold, in the neighborhood of 30 degrees. I was sitting next to a Coxswain on the port side of the crew's mess when a plate of breakfast including baked beans came flying across the mess compartment just between our heads and smashed against the skin of the ship. We both ignored it and kept eating.

At 15 knots, standard cruising speed for "Man-of War" vessels in 1940, the normal transit time from U.S. West coast ports was seven days. As we got nearer the Hawaiian Islands the seas became calm. On the morning of what would have commenced our eighth day at sea, I was presented with one of the most beautiful sights ever when I first went on deck. The island of Oahu, as we approached the entrance to Pearl Harbor, was absolutely spectacular. I was completely taken by the beauty of the setting before me. By 0900, we had entered the harbor and tied up in a nest of destroyers moored along side the Destroyer Tender USS Dixie, AD-14. Both Burch and I were transferred to the Dixie for further transfer to the USS Detroit. However, it was six days before we were finally sent on The Detroit.

We reported aboard The Detroit about 1400, (2:00 PM) on 2 July 1940 and the ship got under way for Hilo located on the Big Island, Hawaii. We anchored about a half mile off the beach about 0900 the morning of 3 July. Early liberty was granted commencing about 1300 and I was lucky enough to rate going ashore. However, I rode the liberty boat as far as the pier and found myself so sick I never got out of the boat. Upon returning to the ship, I went to the sick bay and they turned me in to a bunk with what in those days they called "Cat Fever". Believe me I was one sick sailor. I was kept in the sick bay for about two days and discharged back to the third division for general duty when my fever subsided, although I was so sick during the following couple days that I could hardly stand on my feet. In those days if you did not have a fever you were not considered to be sick.

Rebel Wells, Boatswain Mate First Class was leading Petty Officer of Third Division to which I was assigned. It was the deck division responsible for all weather decks, hull, and appurtenances between the forward and after superstructures. Anyway, Rebel was one of the Old Salts of which we had twenty or twenty-five in a crew of approximately 550 people, including Flag personnel. When one of these individuals spoke you had better listen and heed. Otherwise you most likely would pick yourself up from the deck with a split lip or bloody nose. They tolerated no equivocation nor lack of action in response to their orders. Believe me they ran a tight ship, but one always knew where one stood with those Old Salts.

I remained in the deck force about two months when an opening in the Fire Control Gang developed and I was recommended as a striker. Thinking I would be going down into the Fire Rooms, it was my big surprise when a Fire Controlman Second Class took me in tow and we climbed up the tripod foremast to an enclosure containing the forward main battery Gun Director and Rangekeeper. He removed the cover from the Rangekeeper and I was dumbfounded at the sight of all the various mechanisms, gears, shafts, and dials. My first thought was, "Herriford you will never be able to understand nor master this stuff".

I took the exam for Seaman First Class, passed and was advanced in rate. Course books for Fire Controlman Third Class were given me and my studies began. My battle station became Operator for the Altimeter, a coincidence rangefinder situated on a mount that positioned the line of sight in a slant plane for ranging on aircraft. Following that, I became operator for Main Battery Rangefinder No. 2, located in the after superstructure. It was here, during a short range battle practice, that I first observed two 6-inch projectiles kiss that had been fired from one of our 6-inch twin mounts. Following this gunnery practice, delay compensators were installed in the firing circuits of the left gun in each of the two 6-inch twin mounts causing the left gun to fire 6 milliseconds after the right gun. These twin gun mounts were enclosed in 3/4 inch steel plate housings resembling a turret.

In the spring of 1941, I was ordered to the Elementary Fire Control School at the Destroyer Base, (now the Naval Station) in San Diego, California for a three month course of instruction in Gun Fire Control. My transportation back to the States was in the new fleet tanker USS Santee, AO-29, which took me to Long Beach, California. The Santee would later be converted to an escort aircraft carrier, CVE-29 during the early part of WW-II.

At this time Captain Byron C. McCandless was the commanding officer of the Destroyer Base. As such, he made a deal with the Navy Department that for 10 cents a day per man more ration money, the Destroyer Base therefore using naval personnel, would refurbish all the old 4-stack destroyers moored in the south bay. While the various schools were not involved in the destroyer effort, let me tell you we ate like kings since everyone shared the same mess hall.

While in school, it was mandatory that all students be assigned duty on the base watch list. The normal four hour watches were split such that only half the watch standers available were on watch at one time. The other half were on standby but permitted to relax in the old mess hall where night rations were available. One night when I had the mid-watch the Captain came into the mess hall about 0200 and observed the 8 or 10 standbys with nothing to do. He therefore took several hands across the street to a tool shed, broke out some hoes, shovels, and rakes along with a wheelbarrow and had the standby section of the watch policing up the area in the middle of the night.

Captain McCandless was a very eccentric old cuss, but along with all that, he was very proud of his accomplishments on the Base. He was known to dress in dungarees from time to time. One story was that a sailor with a sea bag on his shoulder approached the ladder going aboard the old USS Regal which, at that time served as both the Receiving Ship as well as the Commanding Officers Quarters and asked the individual standing nearby, "Hey, Pop—give me a hand with my sea bag". The individual so addressed assisted and once aboard enlightened the sailor that he was addressing the Commanding Officer. The Captain was so proud of the food served in the crew's mess that, dressed in dungarees, he was known to come through the mess line and eat with the men on occasion.

Following completion of school in San Diego, I was transported via destroyer back to light cruiser Detroit in Pearl Harbor the latter part of June 1941. I was advanced to the rate of Fire Controlman Third Class, (FC/3c) on 1 August 1941.

From the very first time I arrived in Pearl Harbor, liberty was restricted to midnight, if you were stationed aboard a ship, (Cinderella Liberty). This applied to all hands, except Officers, Chief Petty Officers and a few Petty Officers First Class who were lucky enough to have their wives in Honolulu. In those days it was forbidden for Ensigns and any one below the rate of Petty Officer Second Class to be married. Imagine ten thousand sailors descending on Honolulu on Saturday and again on Sunday. Except for Woo Fats restaurant, Hotel Street was simply one bar after another. Numerous bordellos occupied the side streets. Among them were names like The New Senator and Honolulu Rooms. When ten to fifteen thousand sailors hit the beach in Honolulu on a Saturday or Sunday there were only two things for 95 percent of them to do. For three dollars, they could get a lay in one of the cathouses and or they could consume their fair share of booze in a bar. Remember the novel "Marrie Stover"?

By now, the situation with Japan was beginning to look pretty grim. All during the summer of 1941, the Pacific Fleet held numerous exercises including both day and night maneuvers every time we put to sea. It seems to me that we spent about two out of three weeks of our time at sea, although we usually entered Pearl Harbor on a Friday afternoon and put to sea again on Monday morning. Usually we would remain in port for routine upkeep one week out of every three. Emergency drills were conducted almost every day whether in port or at sea. Later during the Attack on Pearl Harbor, I recall being very thankful for all those drills, when I was to observe how all hands responded to that emergency. To my knowledge, not a single man shirked his duty and in many instances our training was such that if a vacancy was observed, the first individual on the scene filled the spot until the assigned crewmember arrived. I observed acts of super human effort that morning that absolutely defies imagination. Later, people involved in these efforts were unable to repeat the feats.

One such occasion involved a torpedoman's striker. This individual weighed in at 115 pounds at most. Yet, during the attack he made numerous trips down to group four magazine, shouldered a box of four rounds of 3 inch ammunition weighing 134 pounds, then climbing up 3 deck levels and delivered the ammo to one of the AA guns approximately 150 feet from the hatch. Sometime after the attack several people tried to get this individual to repeat the feat and he could not even so much as lift one of those 4-round boxes of 3" ammunition.

Commencing in August of 1941, live ammunition was stowed in the ready service boxes 24 hours a day, at sea or in port. I recall burlap bags draped over the ready service boxes with a fire hose dribbling water to wet the burlap to keep the stowages cool. This became routine until Detroit had to enter the floating dry dock for emergency repairs to our screws. At this time ready service ammunition was secured below decks in the magazines. We entered the floating dry dock on Monday morning and left it on Friday morning 5 December 1941. Detroit put to sea that morning for speed trials following repairs to the engineering plant. This was a mandated requirement to make maximum full throttle speed for a period of 4 hours. Normally speed of the ship will not be divulged during a speed run. Being a Fire Controlman, ships speed is of concern to the solution of the Fire Control Problem, therefore, I made a point of inquiring. All I got from the Quartermaster of the watch was that we were exceeding 36 knots. When we returned to Pearl Harbor late the afternoon of 5 December, live ammunition was not again brought out of the magazine and stowed in the ready service boxes at the AA gun locations. Detroit moored in F-13, her normally assigned berth, the furthermost inland on the Pearl City side of Ford Island.

8

Pearl Harbor: Untold Events

Through the years, following the attack on Pearl Harbor, there has been little or nothing written, to my knowledge, of events involving the light cruiser USS Detroit, CL-8 which, transpired both during the attack and the week following.

This writer was in the "F" Division, comprised of people responsible for the operational readiness of all offensive weapons systems within the ship. I was a Fire Controlman Third Class, (FC/3c) and my battle station was Operator of Main Battery Rangefinder #1. Upon commencement of the attack, I had just sat down to breakfast when a loud thump was felt followed several seconds later by another such sound. Someone made the remark that a boat coxswain would certainly get chewed out by the Officer of the Deck, (OOD) for bumping his boat against the ship. However, a Chief Gunners Mate passing through the mess area happened to look out through a port and exclaimed, "It's the Japs, this is the real thing." The General Alarm immediately sounded calling all hands to battle stations. I dropped the spoon of cereal without taking a single bite of breakfast and dashed for my battle station. Proceeding up through hatch number one on my way to the rangefinder, I recall seeing someone who had just missed being strafed, hunkered behind the port leg of the tripod Foremast for protection.

Range-One was situated one deck level above the Pilot House. A twenty-four inch signal light mounted on a platform approximately eighteen inches above the deck atop the pilot house must be crossed in order to proceed higher into the forward superstructure. I was on the signal light platform when Vulmer Dates, who was squatted down behind the Rangefinder base, yelled at me to duck. Immediately I jumped and dived into the Rangefinder housing while Dates followed. With both of us inside the shield, I activated the instrument. Our forward 3 inch AA gun, located on the centerline forward and one deck level below the pilot house, fired several rounds in an aft direction and the concussion popped covers off the ports on either side of the Rangefinder housing. All at once, after having looked out through the port on his side, Dates leaned over against me with index fingers in both ears. I asked him what the problem was. There was no answer for some period of time. Finely removing his fingers he glanced out the port again then remarked to me "That was the biggest damned torpedo I have ever seen". Apparently a torpedo bomber approaching from the direction of Pearl City had been foiled from dropping his fish by concentrated fire from our eight 50 Caliber machine guns.

We had been inside the Rangefinder just a few minutes when we exited and looked around. The first thing we noticed was two trails across the deck showing 6 or 8 bright shining steel spots in each trail surrounded by red-lead in the gray deck surface. Here was evidence that Dates, having yelled at me to duck, had saved me from being strafed. We observed the Jap plane that crashed into the USS Curtis as it was taken under fire by both cruisers USS Detroit and USS Raleigh, and we were looking directly at the USS Arizona when she exploded. At first we thought it was a fuel tank over behind the Submarine Base, but immediately observed it to be one of our battleships. There was the corona of a shock-wave observed, but I do not recall hearing a loud report, just a slight rush of air a few seconds following the explosion.

The level of Range-One was approximately 65 feet above the water line. Therefore, Dates and I had a pretty clear view of the entire harbor, with nothing to do, except watch the destruction. The uniform of the day was white shorts and "T" shirts and although we were in the tropics, I recall being extremely cold. I was actually shivering. Had I been one iota more scared I believe I would have dropped dead on the spot.

We observed geysers of water 4 and 5 times higher than the fighting tops of the battleships along battleship row each time a torpedo struck one of them. Those fighting tops were approximately 135 feet above the water line. We watched the battleship USS Nevada get underway and steam past the carnage along the length of battleship row, and observed numerous Jap planes swarm over her as she made her way toward Hospital Point. Considering the damage she had suffered, she was intentionally run aground to prevent blocking the channel…The destroyer USS Shaw, in the floating dry-dock, made a spectacular sight as her forward magazines exploded, blowing off her entire bow and bridge superstructure forward of her forward stack. Fourth of July fireworks were never more spectacular.

By this time, both Dates and I were in a state of shock. I, therefore requested permission to secure the Rangefinder and go below to assist on the AA battery, the idea being it would give us something to do. The request was denied along with instructions to keep Range-One manned, that we were making ready to get under way. Range-One was normally manned during Special Sea Detail in order to provide navigational ranges while entering or leaving port. Little did we know that it would be approximately 30 hours later before we would secure from general quarters.

A torpedo had missed our stern by about 10 feet and ran upon the beach at Ford Island, less than 200 feet from the ship. This occurred during the first phase of the attack. The second phase consisted primarily of high level bombing during which, two sticks of bombs narrowly missed the ship and deposited mud from the harbor bottom on some of our weather decks. About 0945 the attacking forces withdrew. We were very lucky in that having been strafed from stem to stern, missed by attempted torpedoing on at least two occasions, and further missed by the horizontal bombing, only one person was wounded when a machine gun bullet went through the fleshy part of his thigh and the ship sustained only superficial damage.

During the early part of the attack I recall glancing down onto the starboard wing of the bridge and observing Rear Admiral Milo F. Draemel, Commander Destroyers Battle Force, (COMDESBATFOR) issuing orders to various of his staff officers for the orderly getting under way of destroyers under his command. Scared as I was it was reassuring to me to note the calm demeanor of the Admiral and his staff, almost as if it was routine.

Detroit got under way at 1010 hours, without benefit of tugs, from our usual berth at F-13. Normally we utilized two tugs for mooring or getting under way. Rather than circle Ford Island as we usually did, we turned the ship around in Eastlock, on the Pearl City side of the harbor, to avoid having to pass along battleship row in the process of leaving the harbor. It was about the time we got under way that Dates and I first noticed our sister cruiser USS Raleigh, CL-7 moored at berth F-12 astern of us exhibiting a very severe list to port. Her crew was busy stripping ship. Already her catapults had been dumped over the side and all mooring lines she had on board had been broken out and passed between the ship and quays. We also noted that USS Utah moored astern of Raleigh had capsized. Dense smoke and fire was observed all along the other side of Ford Island along battleship row, in the vicinity of the sea plane ramps and hangers as well as in the dry dock area of the Navy Yard.

After completing our turn-around, Detroit was ordered to return to our berth at F-13. We tied up port side to on orders from Commander and Chief U.S. Pacific Fleet (CinCPAC). Rear Admiral Draemel was made Commander Task Force One with orders to investigate possible landing of Japanese forces along the western beaches on the island of OAHU, our island, and thereafter seek out and engage attacking forces. When again we got under way to leave the harbor, as we passed Raleigh, her ships company, most of whom were topside yelled all kinds of remarks like "Go get those dirty little yellow, sneaky sons-of-bitches", etc. The light cruiser USS St. Louis left the harbor just ahead of Detroit. Both ships steamed out through the channel about noon or maybe a little before doing about 20 knots. A speed unheard of during normal circumstances, but considered necessary for fear of torpedo attack as we excited the channel.

Sure enough, Detroit, under the command of Capt. L.J. Wiltse, USN was no sooner clear of the channel when a patrolling destroyer sent a blinker light message that two torpedoes were heading toward us. Captain Wiltse took evasive action and some eight or ten minutes later two end of run detonations were observed on the horizon. Investigation disclosed no landings in progress on Oahu, so Task Force One formed up and commenced a search for the attacking forces. The smoking lamp was lit in restricted safe areas in mid-afternoon and both Dates and I each lighted cigarettes from burning $20.00 bills, which we had in turn set afire with our cigarette lighters. We figured this was a one-way trip. However, the old "Gentleman" up above must have been looking down on us with kind thoughts, otherwise I would not be writing this.

9

Post Attack Operations

Late in the afternoon of the 7th, we formed up with several other ships. The task force commander sent various destroyers fanning out in different directions, scouting for some sign of the attackers. About midnight when everything was so very quiet, I overheard the Admiral remark, "Give them another 10 seconds to identify themselves, then if they do not, open fire". Almost immediately, I distinguished a blinker light message being sent to us. There was what could be discerned as a sigh of relief down on the bridge. Apparently both Dates and I had dozed off for a short time before the conversation down on the bridge alerted us. This scared the hell out of me. I could see us being shot for sleeping on watch. Later in the wee hours of the morning, I really got a jolt when the Chief Fire Controlman banged on the shield doors to wake us up. It seemed Forward Control could not raise us on the sound powered battle telephone circuit. Most everyone was exhausted and I later learned people were cat-napping every chance they got. We had been at General Quarters continuously for about 18 hours without food or water.

Somehow, we got through the night and about mid-morning sandwiches and hot coffee were distributed. I recall taking a wonderful looking ham sandwich and a cup of hot coffee, but it was all I could do to force down a single bite and a single sip. The rest I gave to someone else who apparently was not in the state of shock I seemed to be in.

Our task force rendezvoused with the aircraft carrier USS Enterprise task group the afternoon of the 8th. This combined force searched the quadrant South to West of the Hawaiian Islands until Wednesday, 10 December without any sign of Japanese forces. USS Detroit returned to Pearl on the afternoon of the 10th to a sight that almost turned my stomach. Oil and debris of various descriptions were to be found pretty well all over the harbor. Blackened ships having various degrees of list were sitting on the harbor bottom, or capsized, or exhibiting a horrible mass of wreckage, along with burned and wrecked aircraft and hangers were a terrible sight to behold.

We tied up starboard side to our usual berth, F-13. It was noted that a salvage ship, a floating crane and several pontoons were secured around the Raleigh, and her list had considerably lessened. The Special Sea Detail was secured somewhere around 1500 to 1600 hours. I am not sure of the exact time, although all hands were ordered to off-load all target ammunition, to be replaced with service ammunition and to take on fuel oil, stores and provisions. In all my naval career I have never seen an all hands evolution that ever came close to matching this. All hands including all junior officers commenced work with vigor. The evening meal was served in two shifts, so that work at hand was continued without interruption.

I was in the first shift to eat. About half way through someone topside dropped an inert six-inch target projectile on the steel deck. Without exception, every man on the mess deck who had been sitting down at a mess table, simultaneously bolted upright to a standing position, resulting in a very loud clatter of mess benches tipping over throughout the mess spaces. Just an example of fragmented nerves and state of shock.

This meal was the first food of any amount to speak of I had consumed since the previous Saturday evening when ashore in Honolulu. Although very delicious looking sandwiches, fruit and coffee were brought around to our various battle stations the morning of the 8th, I found myself in such a state of shock it was impossible to swallow any-thing I attempted to eat. My appetite was just beginning to return as I sat down to this meal. A trip to the Sick Bay to step on the scales revealed I had lost 10 pounds in the three an a half days since the attack.

We worked throughout the night in blacked out conditions taking on fuel, stores, provisions, and ammunition. Actually, these efforts con-tinued well into the following day, 11 December. All items that were not essential to the efficient operation of the ship were sent ashore.

Approximately mid-day on Thursday, 11 Dec, several people spotted a periscope bearing down on the port side of the ship. Some contended it was a swab-handle floating in the water. However, a couple small boats were sent to investigate. One of our motor launches put a grapnel hook over the side and soon found it was being towed stern first about the harbor by that "swab handle". Having observed all this, Captain Wiltse ordered all hands not on duty to lay over to the starboard side of the ship. This threat was identified as another two-man Japanese sub-marine that had somehow gained entrance to the harbor. Apparently at least two of them had come into the harbor early the morning of the 7th rather than only one that has been so stated over the years. During the balance of the afternoon and evening all hands were ordered to the starboard side of the ship on several occasions when this two man sub approached the ship to port. Throughout the night, the sub was held at bay by a number of our small boats and many lookouts with the aid of hand lanterns.

On Friday morning, 12 Dec, three motorboats from the battleships arrived on scene. During the previous night, a Warrant Officer devised and installed crude underwater listening equipment in them. About 0900 hours RADM Draemel ordered a PT boat to come along side. A 2 x 4 was nailed across the stern of the PT with a couple lengths of white line secured underneath. The PT was then sent to a four stack destroyer where two 300 pound depth charges were obtained. When a plot of the suspected sub position was obtained from data provided by the listening motorboats, the PT would then make a run on the designated spot, whereupon a sailor sitting on his butt with feet pushing against the ashcan, would on command throw the white lines over the stern and kick the depth charge over the stern with his feet. The PT had to utilize its power and speed to get clear of the explosion.

Later a second PT was called into similar service, except it employed two 600 pound depth charges obtained from one of our newer destroyers. These depth charge operations continued until late in the afternoon of Friday 12 Dec. It was then determined that the sub had exhausted most of its oxygen supply and had settled to the harbor bottom under the hospital ship USS Solace.

On Saturday morning, 13 Dec, tugs towed the Solace broadside over to the next pair of mooring buoys. The large floating crane was brought to the area along with a lighter/barge. Divers descended, secured lines around the two-man sub and it was lifted up onto the lighter/barge. Thus, the attack on Pearl Harbor finally ended. Whatever happened to the sub, and it's crew members, (if alive) have never been divulged. Many people are of the opinion that only one two-man sub got into the harbor however, this event accounts for at least two. This accounts for the fourth sub, which has to this point never been accounted for in any verbal or written material I have been privy to.

The 2-man subs thus accounted for are first the one sunk by the USS Ward off the entrance to Pearl Harbor. The second was the one which ran ashore off Wheeler Field. The third entered the harbor and was put out of action when the USS Curtis put a 5 inch round through it's coming tower. The fourth 2-man sub was that involved in the action described above. As for the fifth sub, I have never heard of any accounting for this unit.

10

Convoy Duty

On Saturday afternoon, the 13th, my division officer, Lt. Thompson arranged for me to have four hours ashore to look for two second cousins, Jack and Mike Branson. They were stationed aboard the battleship USS West Virginia. It took considerable talking by me to convince Mr. Thompson that this was very important to me as well as to my Uncle who was also my shipmate aboard Detroit, that being Al Herriford. The West Virginia had taken six or more torpedoes and was sitting on the harbor bottom in battleship row. It took me most of the afternoon, but I finally acquired good news concerning both Jack and Mike Branson. Neither had suffered any physical wounds. Jack was engineer in the captain's Gig and Mike was mess cooking when the attack started. Jack's boat was very busy running people between the fleet landing and various ships. Mike, on the other hand, was forced to hand walk a line passed between the main masts of his ship and the USS Tennessee in order to escape fire on the water surrounding the ships. Jack had been transferred to the heavy cruiser New Orleans and Mike to the heavy cruiser Salt Lake City.

In the process of tracking down information on the Branson brothers, I went through the Naval Hospital looking for them. The sight of all the wounded men was appalling. I was especially taken by the sight of a ship's cook from the battleship USS Nevada, with whom I had had a few drinks in a bar in Honolulu on the night of 6 December. He was lying on a bed set up on a verandah, partially covered with a sheet. Both

Legs however, were uncovered with no bandages and the sight nearly turned my stomach. His name I do not recall, but he looked delirious and I walked on past without trying to make conversation.

Having taken on board fuel, ammunition, and all the food and provisions we could possible find storage for, USS Detroit was confined to Pearl Harbor awaiting orders. On December 18, 1941 we got under way about 0800. Upon exiting the harbor, we joined two old four pipe and two more modern destroyers after which, two large liner type ships coming out of Honolulu harbor steamed into our formation. One of the transports was the SS Lurline of the Matson Lines. The other was the SS President Coolidge loaded with evacuees, i.e. wives and families of both military personnel and civilians employed by the military as well as construction firms were being returned to continental U.S. The Lurline, still wearing her beige colored paint was loaded with wounded from the Pearl Harbor Attack. The formation assumed a zigzag course for San Francisco at 15 knots.

Many years later, in 1953, Jaretta, Shirley, (my wife and daughter) and I became neighbors of Fred, Fran and their son Fred McMillan, Jr. at the Naval Ordnance Test Station, China Lake, California. We became very close friends and I then learned that Fran and Fred Jr. were both passengers in the President Coolidge on that fateful cruise back to the States.

Two old 4-stack destroyers stayed with us throughout the first day and night. About 0900 the second day they turned 180 degrees and returned to Pearl Harbor. From there on, USS Detroit, the two newer destroyers and two transports proceeded to San Francisco. On the morning of 25 December 1941 this formation of 5 ships steamed under the Golden Gate Bridge, the first ships to return from Pearl Harbor since the attack. Word of our arrival spread all around the Bay area like wildfire.

Detroit anchored out in the bay adjacent to Yerba Buena, (Goat) Island and west of the Bay Bridge. About a 2 mile boat ride from the Ferry Building in San Francisco. Liberty was granted at 1300 hours, (1:00 PM), and it was my good fortune to be in the Starboard watch, the first section permitted to go ashore. The first thing I did was to go to the Western Union office at 3rd and Broadway and send a telegram home to Granddad and Grandmother Herriford that both Al and I along with Jack and Mike Branson were all safe and well. The idea being that they would in turn notify everyone else including my mother in Tulsa. I learned much later that this was the first positive word any-one back home had of the status of we four boys

Next, I drifted up to the tenderloin section and went into the Streets of Paris. This was a bar I had frequented on previous trips to San Fran-cisco. Lo and behold, sitting at one of the nearest tables to the door was a snipe, (Fireman) from the ship. With him were two women and they invited me to join them. We had several drinks and made small talk. These two ladies were from Sacramento. They were in San Francisco on business and heard about Detroit being in port, so decided to spread a little cheer to some of her sailors. However, they had to leave us to take care of their business, but made a date to meet us that evening at 2000, (8:00 PM). When they again joined us, the one I paired off with bought me a toothbrush and a fifth of White Horse scotch. Following that we had dinner and the women picked up the tab. Then they took us to their hotel where they had a suite of rooms. The balance of the night was spent making whoopee. The Fireman, (I do not remember his name) and I were supposed to catch a boat at the Ferry Building back to the ship at 0600 next morning. Our lady friends took us down to the boat landing by taxi and again picked up the fare. Fog was so heavy the boats could not run, so we had breakfast in a coffee shop and whiled away the time until about 1000 when the fog lifted. The last we saw of the two ladies was their waving as our boat pulled away from the dock. The Port section was granted liberty commencing at 1300. Expiration of liberty the following morning was 0600. Not a single person was absent and the ship got under way about 0800.

Detroit passed under the Golden Gate Bridge and many eyes looked up and wondered if they would be lucky enough to pass under this bridge again. Every time it was my experience to exit the Golden Gate during the war, these thoughts came to mind. 27 December 1941 was no exception. A convoy of twenty-one merchant ships assembled off the Farallon Islands just outside the Golden Gate, escorted by Detroit and four or five destroyers. Four or five of these merchantmen were old four-masted steamers of pre-World War-I vintage that used to ply up and down the Pacific coast loaded with lumber. They could make 6 knots, wind and tide in their favor. The cruise to Pearl Harbor took 21 uneventful and monotonous days.

It was very interesting to take note of the deck load on the various ships. One of the old lumber steamers was loaded with Irish potatoes in hundred pound crates filling both holds and stacked on the weather deck to the level of the pilot house. Another two were loaded with lumber stacked to the level of the pilot house also. A couple more modern C3 hulls each had deck loads of 8 or 10 salvage pontoons. Several other ships carried deck loads of heavy construction vehicles. Then there was 5 or 6 tankers loaded with various types of refined petroleum products. When we arrived in the Hawaiian Islands on 17 January 1942, our escorting destroyers fuel supply had almost been reduced to fumes.

USS Detroit refueled, re-provisioned and remained in Pearl Harbor but just a few days. Then we were underway again. This time besides Detroit there were two destroyers and two transports. One of the transports was the four stack HMS Aquatania, sister ship of the HMS Lusatania. The other ship was a twin stack vessel, the Army transport

General Scott. The five ship formation set a course to San Francisco at twenty three knots. No zig zagging. Approximately 77 hours later the transports, and two destroyers passed under the Golden Gate Bridge.

Detroit was still at sea however, searching for one of her scout-observation sea planes. This aircraft was catapulted from Detroit to scout ahead of the convoy for any enemy activity the second day at sea. Toward mid-afternoon, radio signals from the plane were received to the effect they were lost and could not find the formation. For Detroit to break radio silence was out of the question, although we did leave the convoy formation and started making smoke in hopes they would see it. Finally the plane radioed they was low on fuel and going to set down on the ocean surface. The sea was reasonably calm. The search continued until approximately noon the following day.

Because of wartime conditions Detroit could not remain a target for Jap submarines any longer, and the search was abandoned. Perhaps the hardest thing we encountered to this point in the war was to lose two of our crew who were highly respected by all who knew them. The pilot loved to fly and was outstanding the way he handled his airplane. His radioman and observer was an Aviation Machinist Mate 1/c who was highly regarded both as a radioman and observer. Neither they nor their airplane were ever found.

For the next few months Detroit escorted several convoys between Pearl Harbor and San Francisco. We found ourselves in San Francisco more than any other port during the first six months of 1942, although most of our time was spent at sea. Generally we moored in the China Basin area of the waterfront. I was designated Guard Mail Petty Officer and as such found myself going all over San Francisco and boarding numerous ships along the waterfront.

I carried a regular leather U.S. Mail pouch over my shoulder, wore a "Guard Mail" brassard on my left arm and carried a Navy 45 caliber automatic pistol for side arm.

Initially, I was told I could ride the public transportation free. However, on the second day, I boarded a streetcar on Market Street and the conductor threatened to through me off for not paying. After some discussion he still insisted I pay or get off. My patience by now was growing thin, so I let him know in no uncertain terms that he was not about to put me off. Upon returning to the ship, I reported this incident to my superiors and thereafter was provided tokens for fare.

In early March while in Pearl Harbor, I returned to the ship from a guard mail trip to find the submarine USS Trout moored between Detroit and F-13 Quay. Gold ingots of two sizes were being taken aboard ship from the sub along with many sacks of silver pesos and several trunks of negotiable securities, all belonging to the Philippine Government. There must have been about 80 large yellow gold ingots and 30 red gold ingots approximating a third the size of the yellow gold ingots. Altogether, there must have been something like 20 or 25 million dollars worth of treasure to be taken back to the States for safekeeping. When we arrived in San Francisco, Detroit moored to pier 56 in the China Basin near the third Street draw bridge. A Mayflower van backed up to our brow escorted by a couple jeeps loaded with marines, carrying Thompson sub-machine guns. Upon opening up the van, several more marines stepped out also well armed. The van was a bobtail of approximately 2 1/2 tons in size. Two trips were required to transport the gold, silver and securities to the mint for safe keeping.

On one occasion, the ship was scheduled to be in port for two weeks. Until now I had been in the Navy over two years and had never taken a leave. During the war, leave was forbidden, except for survivors who had had ships shot out from under them. Anyway, I was told I could take 10 days leave during the ships two weeks upkeep period. Next it was cut to one week, then to 5 days. Still I was able to get the 5 days plus the weekend.

The result of it all was that I rode a train back to Oklahoma, spent one day visiting my mother in Tulsa, then went to Cleveland to visit my paternal Grandparents for a day and boarded a train back to San Francisco. I reported back aboard ship late on Sunday afternoon, having departed the previous Monday morning.

On one of our convoy trips between Pearl Harbor and San Francisco, we had a medical doctor for a passenger. It had been my misfortune to develop an eye condition that was like granulated eyelids. Our ship's doctor was aware of my problem and asked our passenger who was an eye specialist to have a look at me. He gave a diagnosis of a disease among Indians in Oklahoma. Having originated from Oklahoma, I was to later conclude misdiagnoses of my problem. This passenger doctor recommend painting my eyelids with copper sulfate dipped in sterile water.

On the return trip to Pearl Harbor, again with Detroit escorting a convoy, the ships doctor decided it would be a good time to treat my eyes. The operation turned out to be very painful. Each time the wetted copper sulfate was touched to my eyelids it felt like red hot drops of iron being dropped onto them. Afterward, it felt like both my eyes were full of sand and extremely painful. I was blind for the next three weeks, and confined to the sick bay until we returned to San Francisco. Detroit was scheduled for a month availability in the Mare Island Naval Shipyard, although our doctor transferred me to Treasure Island for further transfer to the Naval Hospital at Mare Island as soon as we arrived in the bay. By the time I arrived at the hospital, the ship was already there.

Anyway, I was kept in the hospital for two weeks during which time my sight slowly began returning. The correct diagnosis was rendered: My initial condition was diagnosed as Bacterial Conjunctivitis, (Pink-eye) that following the treatment using copper sulfate became Chemical Conjunctivitis. The ship still had two weeks of her yard availability left when I returned aboard. I was just beginning to see reasonably well wearing very dark glasses providing I was not in sunlight. Altogether it took approximately six-months for my eyes to get their strength back.

Detroit escorted another convoy to Pearl Harbor upon leaving the shipyard. It was on the way west that I received notice, in the mail taken aboard prior to our departure, to report to my draft board. Well, as it turned out I did not report and to this day I have never had a draft number.

Upon arrival in Pearl Harbor, Jack Branson, my cousin, who was now assigned to the heavy cruiser USS New Orleans, CA-32, formerly of the USS West Virginia, came over to Detroit for a visit. This was the first time we had seen one another since before the attack on Pearl Harbor. He looked fine, but I was still recuperating from my eye problem. Our visit lasted for a couple hours after which, he left the ship and we did not see one another again until after WW-II ended.

This was the early days of June 1942. Ships were entering and leaving Pearl Harbor like I had never seen before. There were rumors about of an impending large naval action in the near future. The night of 4 June, Detroit took aboard a passenger who was berthed in the admiral's quarters. This individual was not identified for some time. He was being returned to the Continental U.S. for treatment of a severe skin condition that to this point no one in the Pacific had been successful in treating. On the morning of 5 June, Detroit again left Pearl Harbor escorting another convoy to the West Coast. This was the day the battle of Midway began. Again this trip was as usual, uneventful. After our arrival in San Francisco it was learned that our passenger on this trip was none other than Admiral William F. (Bull) Halsey famous commander of the Third Fleet.

11

South Pacific

Detroit escorted a convoy out of Pearl Harbor heading for the South Pacific transporting either the Third or Fifth Marine Division, I cannot remember which. There were approximately twelve ships in the formation, nearly all troop transports. We took them as far as Pago Pago, (Pronounced: Pango Pango) Samoa on the island of Tutuila. Detroit turned the convoy over to other U.S. Navy warships which continued on toward the southwest pacific. Entering the harbor at Pago Pago, Detroit refueled. We remained in port two days and got underway for our return trip to Pearl Harbor. Detroit was steaming alone on a zig zag course.

A couple days before our scheduled arrival at Pearl Harbor, about mid-morning, a PBY-5 flying boat flew over us and sent a blinker message providing coordinates where another PBY had developed engine trouble and had set down on the surface. Detroit altered course and went to flank speed. We steamed for ten hours at 32 knots and arrived at the seaplane about an hour before sundown. Thirteen men were aboard, a double crew on a training flight. A small boat was put in the water and took the end of a tow line which was secured to the flying boat, then returned to the ship with the thirteen aircrewmen. Upon getting underway, the ship was very cautious in taking the seaplane in tow. Speed was slowly built up until at about 5 knots the PBY nosed over as if trying to dive. This was a brand new seaplane. The ship stopped and it became apparent we could not tow this beast. Therefore it was sunk using our 20mm guns.

Pearl Harbor was about 300 miles distant, so we steamed on a course during the night that brought us to the channel entrance about 0900 the following morning. When the special sea detail was called to man stations, I got a big surprise as I went onto the weather deck through number one hatch. Standing next to the port leg of the tripod foremast was John Hudsonpiller, the eldest son of the postman who delivered mail on the east side of Cleveland, Oklahoma, my home town of twenty-five hundred souls. We had gone to high school together. A small world, even in those days. I never saw him again.

From Pearl Harbor we proceeded to San Diego. On liberty there I was making my way around the Plaza to ascertain which street car to catch out to my Uncle Maurice and Aunt Pauline's when I heard someone say "Hey". Upon turning around, I looked my dad Square in the face. He was awaiting the same streetcar as I. The last knowledge I had of Dad he was in Oklahoma. His reason for coming to California," he was tired of working all summer to pay last winter's fuel bill". We found Maurice in a bar down town and the three of us proceeded to get plastered. About mid-night Maurice went home and Dad and I retired to his hotel room. Neither of us was feeling any pain.

Dad set the alarm for five O'clock, because I had to be back aboard ship by 0600. The ship was scheduled to get underway at 0800 for the Hunters Point Naval Shipyard in south San Francisco to commence a 30 day availability. When the alarm went off, I managed to get up and dress. However, upon exiting the bathroom I discovered that I had put Dad's kahki shirt on underneath my uniform jumper. Feeling hung over as we were, both of us had a good laugh about the incident. Suffice it to say, I made it back to the ship by 0600

While at Hunters Point our steam radiator heating system was over-hauled. Of all the stupid things, brass fittings were used to couple the steel tubing to the steam lines. This was not discovered until about a month later when the system was needed and failed. More about this later.

After leaving the shipyard, we escorted the 5th Marine Division I believe it was from San Diego to Pago Pago, Samoa. This convoy comprised ten or twelve ships plus Detroit. Again we spent a couple days in port after refueling before heading back to the States.

The channel, about 2 miles long into Pago Pago harbor, was dredged through a reef. The water was sufficiently clear that one could see the coral bottom on either side of the channel. It was through this passage that I became nearest to ever being seasick during my entire naval career. We got underway about 1300, (1:00 PM). I had the afternoon watch in Forward Main Battery Control in the foretop of the tripod mast about 100 feet above the water line. The swells across the reef caused a strange roll and pitch to the ship while in the channel. Being so high in the superstructure further accented the sensation. After clearing the channel and getting into deep water, the ship settled down and things became normal.

There was no convoy to contend with on our return to the States. We set a course for San Francisco to pass just north of the Marquesas Islands. It was in this vicinity that we went to general quarters about 0300 one morning. Our radar had disclosed several ships on a course opposite ours. We challenged them and were within ten seconds of opening fire with our 6 inch 53 caliber main battery guns before they gave a favorable response and identified themselves. It turned out the command ship in the formation was USS Raleigh, CL-7, Detroit's sister ship.

From Samoa, we steamed at approximately 23 knots and arrived in San Francisco with nothing but fumes left in our fuel tanks. We docked at a pier west of the ferry building and a fuel barge was along side almost before the Special Sea Detail was secured. Many cardboard boxes were brought aboard from the warehouse on the pier. Four hours later having completed refueling, we were again underway, steaming out through the Golden Gate. This time our course pointed Northwest.

Almost immediately, the boxes that had been brought aboard were opened and foul weather clothing was issued to all hands. Three days later, we tied up to a pier on Kodiak Island, Alaska. In eight days we had traveled from the equator to a place where the average temperature was 29 degrees below zero, Fahrenheit. It was so cold that the lubricant in all gearboxes froze solid. Working in three separate shifts of two or three men each, we opened those gear boxes, removed the frozen lubricant, cleaned the interior of the mechanism and introduced diesel oil for lubrication. This operation had to be performed on all ordnance equipment exposed to the weather. It was necessary to remove our foul weather mittens in order to dismantle and reassemble the equipment. Therefore, working time on station for each shift was limited to ten minutes. While one shift was on station, the one just relieved would go below and peel off their foul weather clothing to get warm while the third shift would be getting into their gear, preparing to go topside to relieve the shift that by now was practically frozen. For ten days, this was the routine for 12 to 14 hours a day.

On one occasion, I did manage to get ashore for about two hours while in Kodiak. Except for lots of snow and very cold weather nothing stands out in my mind, except I recall a very pretty young girl walking down the street dressed in medium brown short fur out side with light gray fur cuffs and parka. What really caught my attention was her bright rosey cheeks, although it was evident she wore no make-up. Detroit left Kodiak the following day.

12

An Epidemic

Detroit left Kodiak and proceeded to Adak, an island about half way out in the Aleutian chain, where the Army Air Corps had established an air base from which P38 fighters and B24 bombers flew. The Navy was also flying PBY-5's from there to navigate for the bombers when they made strikes on Kiska and Attu that had been occupied by the Japs at the time of the battle of Midway. We tied up along side the old fleet tanker USS Brazos from which, we took on some provisions and refueled. Following that, we got under way and proceeded to sea where, we rendezvoused with our sister ship USS Raleigh and four destroyers. Twice more at about one week intervals the entire five ship group entered Adak for replenishment during daylight hours. After that, we always entered Adak after dark and had to be back at sea and over the horizon before daylight. At this point in time, Task Force 16, consisting of light cruisers Detroit, (Flag), Raleigh and four destroyers comprised the major naval force in the Aleutian Island and Bearing Sea area until sometime in January 1943. From November 1942 until March 1943 there were only two days of liberty for the ships company and that was in Dutch Harbor during Christmas. Otherwise we were, for all practical purposes continuously at sea, except for our periodic excursions, normally once a week, into Adak for overnight replenishment.

Soon after our arrival in the outer Aleutian operating area, a case of "Strep Throat" broke out on the ship. Our crew approximated about 780 men and about two thirds of them were afflicted, while about half of those had to be confined to bed. We had two doctors on board. They acquired all the sulfanilamide available from the various ships and the air base at Adak. Later, one of the doctors told me the epidemic was so severe that had it not been for the sulfa drug, half of those affected would have died. It took about ten days to conquer this problem. I was one of the fortunate third of the crew that did not come down with the malady. However, needing some medical tape for a job I was doing, one morning upon entering the dispensary, the doctor stuck a thermometer in my mouth and insisted I take a ration of pills just to be on the safe side. My temperature was below normal, having just come in from the bitter cold outside. .

Remember, this was wintertime in these parts. The average temperature was 34 degrees below zero Fahrenheit throughout the winter. A wind velocity of 35 knots results in a chill factor of approximately-104 degrees. Sometimes the wind velocity was as high as 60 knots with chill factor down to-116 degrees. This is really cold and is especially so when at general quarters on the after main battery gun director, which was the highest point in the after superstructure and completely exposed to the elements. I received frostbites on my chin and right thumb because it was necessary to remove the mouth cover on my facemask and take off my right glove in order to talk on a set of sound powered battle telephones and to stow them upon securing from general quarters. This occurred one night when we went to General Quarters, (GQ) about 0200. The wind was blowing sea spray almost horizontal with the droplets partially frozen by the time they struck.

Whenever Task Group 16 returned to Adak to replenish, it was an all night operation. There was no interruption in the Condition Three watch schedule, (one watch on and two watches off). If not on watch during normal working hours, one really worked. The biggest effort was chipping away the accumulation of twenty some years of paint in the living spaces and below decks compartments that was an extreme fire hazard. My job was altogether different however, thanks to my division officer, Ltjg Parris. For some reason or another, he had a dislike for me. He assigned me the job of fabricating sheet metal chests to replace the wooden spare parts boxes in our ordnance storeroom.

I determined the number of sheets of 16 gauge galvanized steel, hasps, hinges and handles needed and submitted a requisition for the material to be brought on board when we went to Dutch Harbor for Christmas. We remained in Dutch Harbor for three days replenishing and left the day after Christmas. Some of our people went ashore there for two or three hours, but I got no farther than the pier. There was next to nothing in the little village out side the naval base, but some people came by some sort of cheap liquor and managed to sneak it aboard.

I arranged for the C&R shop in the ship to shear and break the sheet metal providing I performed the layout. Ltjg Parris found out about the arrangement and informed me in no uncertain terms, that he intended I was to perform all the fabrication. Keep in mind that we were in the Bearing Sea where waves of twenty and thirty feet were normal with the ship constantly rolling and pitching. Utilizing hand tools only, I proceeded to construct 12 or 14 metal spare parts boxes in the passageway of the living space outside the Fire Control Shop. Surprisingly, they turned out far better than I expected.

Usually after an all night session in Adak, and when we were back out to sea, it was standard practice to pass the word at 0800, "All hands turn to, commence ships work". Detroit was flagship for Rear Admiral McMorris commanding Task Force 16. After about the third or fourth time of this routine, the Admiral approached the ships commanding officer with the remark, "Captain, I have observed these men stand watch, be up all night on all hands evaluations, and put in a full day of work, but I am wondering if they ever get time to sleep". Immediately and thereafter, upon leaving Adak at 0800 the word was passed "all hands not on watch spread bunks at will". The cold weather, rough seas and incessant work were, until this time, resulting in exhaustion for the entire crew. Rough as it was for the cruisers, pity those poor sailors in the destroyers.

On one occasion, we steamed out of Adak in the midst of a vicious storm. Seas were running 70 feet high. Light cruiser USS Raleigh was 500 yards distant on Detroit's starboard beam. Both ships were on the same course. The seas were so high that each ship would completely disappear from sight of one another from time to time. We steamed for seven days and nights on the same course and were within 50 miles of where we started.

Detroit would ride upon a wave and teeter, with150 feet of her bow and 150 feet of her stern out of the water. When those four screws came clear of the water, you had better be holding onto something solid. The vibration was so severe it could knock a person off his feet. I have been up in the forward main battery fire control station and witnessed green water come over the 105 foot foretop. Detroit on one occasion rolled 49 degrees. Damage to the ship as a result of this storm was 57 broken frames, the bottom in the fore part of the ship was caved in 2 1/2 inches, with two buckets of rivets having been popped out and the two after main engines secured because of steam turbine blade failures. The pinion gear shaft became bent such that the forward twin 6-inch gun mount could not be trained in azimuth. I observed 3 inches of frost inside the gun mount housing on one occasion, with the full twin-gun crew on watch inside.

We covered the invasion of Amchitka in early February 1943. Following that, in getting under way from along side the tanker USS Brazos in Adak, a willi-waw, (a sudden vicious wind) caught us forcing our stern into the side of the tanker, cutting a hole in Brazos and shearing our forward starboard screw off up to the hub. Detroit was granted a 30 day emergency yard period in Bremerton, Washington for repairs. Several days later, we steamed into Puget Sound doing 12 knots on one of four engines.

After completing the yard period, Detroit left Bremerton and went to pier 92 in Seattle, where we remained a couple days for replenishment of fuel, stores, and provisions. I had liberty the day before we were to get underway again. I was walking along the pier with a Boatswain Mate 1/c, he all at once turned and waved to the ship and uttered "Good Bye, you old son of a bitch". When I asked what that was all about, he informed me "That old bucket of bolts is going back to the Aleutians, but not me". Sure enough, he was not aboard when we got under way the following morning. I did learn later however, that he turned himself in to the Commandant of the 13th Naval District. Word also trickled back to us that he wound up with shore duty upon reassignment.

The second day out, word was received relative to the battle of The Komandorski Islands. This battle lasted for about 3 hours and 45 Minutes, the longest naval battle in modern history. Our skipper, Captain Gisselman increased speed and we arrived in Adak about 72 hours after the battle had concluded. I did not learn until about 1995, that Detroit's CO at this time, Captain Gisselman, was Executive Officer on the USS Arizona during the attack on Pearl Harbor.

When we left the Aleutians and Bearing Sea area, Task Force 16 Flag was transferred to USS Richmond, CL-9 ten (6-inch/53 Cal) guns, another four-stack light cruiser similar to Detroit. There were ten four-stack cruisers in the Omaha class ships of which these ships belonged.

The heavy cruiser USS Salt Lake City, CA-25, ten (8-inch/55 Cal) guns had also relieved Raleigh. The Richmond and Salt Lake City along with four destroyers, therefore comprised Task Force 16. I am not sure, but I believe the four destroyers were USS Bailey, USS Bancroft, USS Benson, and USS Cogland.

On 26 March 1943, a Japanese force of two heavy cruisers, two light cruisers, and five destroyers were escorting several heavily laden transports to replenish bases on Attu and Kiska when they encountered Task Force 16. Despite being heavily outgunned, the American force under Rear Admiral Charles McMorris in Richmond attacked. The Salt Lake City received several major shell hits, and lost steering control for a period of time. While steaming in circles, the story goes that her Main Battery People were guessing numbers to see which gun would miss out on the final salvo. Having ten guns in her main battery of 8-inch guns she had expended all but 9 rounds. Two of the destroyers and the Richmond laid smoke screens around Salt Lake City while the Bailey along with another destroyer made torpedo runs on the Japanese force. One or more hits were scored and with fires visible on two of the larger ships, Vice Admiral Moshiro Hosogaya broke off the attack and joined his transports in retreat.

By the time Detroit arrived in Adak, the USS Salt Lake City had departed the area bound stateside for some much needed repairs. For us it was back to the old routine, although it was evident several additional ships were on the scene in the Aleutian area.

13

Dutch Harbor to Seattle

On or about 3 May 1943, I was transferred from the Detroit with orders to report to the Commanding Officer, Advanced Fire Control School, Washington, D.C. We were along side the old fleet tanker USS Brazos in Adak, and I was sent aboard her for transportation to Dutch Harbor. Little did I realize at the time, that this would be the last time I would ever see that old bucket of bolts, the USS Detroit, CL-8. This last statement is with much nostalgia for that "Grand Old Lady". She was in Pearl Harbor during the "sneak" attack and she was anchored adjacent to the battleship USS Missouri, BB-63 during the signing of the surrender accords by Japan on 2 September 1945, thus ending World War-II. Except for vessels conducting minesweeping operations, Detroit was one of the first U.S. man-of-war ships to enter Tokyo Bay upon cessation of hostilities. Her mission, to pick up navigation charts at Yokohama for Tokyo Bay and deliver them to U.S. Fleet units off the coast.

When USS Brazos arrived in Dutch Harbor, I transferred to the receiving station awaiting further transfer to the Seattle. There was no semblance of transportation out of Dutch Harbor for several days until the SS Columbia, an ancient passenger liner on the Alaska Lines, came into port. Having nothing to do, I hiked the half mile over to where Columbia was tied up. It came to my attention that both Army and Marine personnel were being taken aboard. Spotting the Chief Purser at the head of the brow, (Gangway) I inquired about the possibility of becoming a passenger, having ascertained the Columbia was bound for Seattle. He informed me that if I could produce a TR, (Transportation Request) he would welcome me aboard.

Prior to my departing the Detroit, I approached the Chief Yeoman about the possibility of some leave while in transit to Washington? He informed me an "ALNav" existed forbidding leave, except under very special circumstances. However, he remarked as I started to turn away, "Don't worry about it". When my orders were finally presented to me, it was all I could do to contain myself upon reading them. They stated as follows: "Upon being detached from your present duty, you will travel via the most direct route of transportation and report to the Commanding Officer Advanced Fire Control School, Washington, D.C." One should note the lack of any dates. More on this subject later.

I hiked back to the Receiving Station and spoke to the personnel officer about acquiring a TR . He was happy to comply and within a couple hours I was aboard the SS Columbia bound for Seattle. Of all the military personnel on board as passengers, I was the only sailor. Both Army and Marine contingents had been brought aboard by Colonels. Therefore, all choice accommodations had been taken. Guess where you know who was berthed? You are right. Steerage was the only available space left.

In addition to all military passengers, there were a hundred or so civilian construction workers, who had completed an air base near Fairbanks, heading back to the States with their pockets loaded.

The first night out, I slept in a canvas bottomed bunk in a 2x4 framework about four or five levels above the deck. Suffice it to say, I was not happy with the prospect of spending the following nine nights in these accommodations. However, to my surprise next morning, the Steerage Purser came to me with a proposal I could not refuse. He had noticed I was the only sailor on the passenger list and felt I should be entitled better treatment than to be lodged in Steerage. His proposal was that I could use the second bunk in his stateroom providing I would assist in the crews mess at mealtime with setting the tables and helping with cleaning up afterward. Furthermore, I would have use of the crew's washing machine to do my laundry, which in turn I could hang in the combination engine and fire room to dry. Also I was given access to a refrigerator containing night rations in addition to having use of the crews head and shower facilities.

There was one other perk that proved most beneficial. The Steerage Steward ran the bingo game. This was one facet of the casino situated in the fore part of the ship, all of which was run by various members of the crew. I was instructed to come play bingo, but to purchase a single card only and not to exchange it for another card. Further, I was told when, (not if) I won a game to get up and leave. Invariably, some where between the first and sixth games I would win a $35.00 or $40.00 pot. That was quite substantial in 1943, when a dollar was a dollar. There was never a question of my not winning. The bingo cards cost fifty cents a game. Upon arriving in Seattle I had acquired approximately $300.00 that came in very handy. However, there was a very sad situation among the civilian construction workers. While most of them were flush with cash when they boarded the Columbia, many of them were flat broke upon their arrival in Seattle.

Columbia tied up in Seattle and all military personnel were ordered to assemble in the warehouse on the pier. Being the only sailor, I fell in with the marines. A Navy Lt. took charge of the marines, but upon viewing my orders, informed me I was on my own and free to go. Therefore I inquired how to get to Com 13, (Commandant 13th Naval District) Headquarters. Within a very few minutes, a cab deposited me in front of a high-rise having all the appropriate nomenclature displayed. Upon checking in with the personnel department, my orders were endorsed and I was issued the necessary Travel Requisitions (TR's) for transportation to Washington, D.C. via Portland, Oregon; Cheyenne; and Chicago.

Before leaving Com 13, I made a point of inquiring as to the starting date of the next class at the Advanced Fire Control School. A good look at my travel itinerary showed that I had 13 days to call my own. After taking the train to Portland where, ordinarily a change of trains was necessary, I purchased a round trip ticket to Oakland, California.

My dad and stepmother were living in Albany, about six miles from Oakland. This was the first time in my naval career of over three years, I really felt like I was on leave. My dad was foreman of the swing shift in a steel plant where mats for aircraft landing strips were being fabricated. My stepmother was manager of the cafeteria at the terminal for Pacific Intermountain Express, (PIE) motor freight lines in Oakland. She also was in the catering business where she was in demand by such individuals as Henry J. Kaiser as well as others of note.

Aside from a good visit with my folks, I managed to live it up for a few days. However, I began to run short of cash. To solve this problem, I worked as a stevedore for three nights unloading a ship of raw sugar at the Sea Island Sugar Mill docks in San Francisco. This was very hard work, but it provided funds for the balance of my leave of 13 days and enough to see me to Washington. Upon returning to Portland, Oregon, I resumed my trip to the letter of my orders, (Via the most direct route of transportation) and arrived a day before the next class started.

There were 36 people in my class consisting of two chief warrant officers, two civilians, about six Chief Fire Controlman, perhaps twenty FC 1/c and the balance was FC 2/c of which, I was one of the latter. Two classes were conducted almost simultaneously. The day class was from 0800 to 1600 and the night class was from 1600 to 2400. The times interchanged every two weeks. Length of course was 33 weeks, during which the Mark 37 Gun Director and 5 inch 38 Caliber dual-purpose guns for a Destroyer Fire Control System were taught. The pace of instruction was very fast. Drop your pencil and you may have missed a very important point in the lecture. After hours study was a must. Upon finishing the course, I was very much surprised at finding myself 4th in a class of 36. One of the big things in my favor was a test score of 100 on the hydraulic power drive for 5-inch 38 Cal guns man-ufactured by General Electric,Co. After this, one of the Chief Warrant Officers started calling me the Whiz Kid. This further resulted in my selection for a two week course of instructor training after which, I was assigned as an instructor at the Fire Control Operators School in Ft. Lauderdale, Florida. During the mid part of the 33-week course, I took the exam for Fire Controlman First Class, (FC/1c) and was advanced in rate. One of the Chief Warrant Officers mentioned above was also ordered to the school in Ft. Lauderdale, although, he remained there for somewhat less than four months when he was ordered elsewhere.

14

Instructor in Fire Control School

About the first week in October 1943, I boarded a train in Washington, D.C. bound for Ft Lauderdale, Florida, with orders to report to the CO at the Fire Control Operators School. My TR called for a Pullman berth. However, upon leaving Jacksonville, Florida the conductor informed me I would have to move forward some 8 or 10 coaches to a chair car. I protested that I had a Pullman berth to Ft. Lauderdale in accordance with my orders and TR, but he ignored me completely and solicited the on board Shore Patrol to insist that I move forward. My predicament was hopeless and I complied. Apparently, some "Snow Bird" had boarded the train in Jacksonville and slipped the conductor some cash and I just happened to be the best candidate for displacement.

The first weekend at my new duty station, I was assigned Shore Patrol. Upon reporting to the permanent Chief Shore Patrolman at the local police station I was made aware that all permanent shore patrolmen, of which there were 6 or 8, were all local cops who had enlisted in the Navy with the proviso that they remain in Ft. Lauderdale. The shore patrol officer, a Ltjg was also a local boy. Later that evening I was appalled when the Chief announced prior to going out on beats that the arrest quota for the evening was 40. I brought this situation to the attention of the CO of the school the following Monday morning, when I requested Captains Mast for this very purpose. However, nothing ever came of it.

A couple months later the newly commissioned destroyer USS Bush, DD-529 put in to Port Everglades on her way to the Pacific. She remained in port 4 or 5 days providing liberty and recreation for her crew. This perhaps would be the last opportunity for such before entering the war zone The morning following their first night of liberty, some 8 or 10 of her crew requested Captains Mast to complain of the treatment they had received from the shore patrol. Most of them were sporting black eyes, split lips, broken noses, etc The Captain had just completed mast when the shore patrol officer drove up to the brow in his station wagon and came aboard with a request to see the CO. He immediately requested the Captain to restrict his men to the ship with no further liberty. The CO was so angry, he had to be restrained by the OOD to keep from throwing the Ltjg over the side. He told the Ltjg to get himself and his vehicle off the pier or he would have his crew do it for him. That evening, the Captain selected the 12 largest people in his ship's compliment and sent them ashore as shore patrolmen and he himself toured the downtown area several times. There was no further problem with the permanent shore patrol while the Bush was in port.

Later, during the height of the "Snow Bird" season many of them commenced complaining to local officials that all military personnel should be prohibited from the downtown area and all beaches, except that immediately fronting the school. This situation got so bad that we at the school rented an old former night club building 5 or 6 miles out northwest of Ft. Lauderdale and established our own club. Transportation was our biggest problem however, until the local Naval Air Station surveyed a small bus, equipped it with 4 used TBM airplane tires and gave it to us. When I left there in June 1945, that club and that vehicle were still being operated by naval personnel.

I instructed a course in stereoscopic optical rangefinder, then was assigned to teach a 6 week course in fire control mathematics. My first math class consisted of 36 students ranging in age from 17 to 44 years. While the 17 year old had not completed high school, several students up in their forties had been out of school for more than 25 years. Then there were 6 or 8 men fresh out of college, who continually bugged me to let them use their slide rules and log tables. The course consisted of simple basic math to begin with up through trigonometry. The final exam being a single antiaircraft problem to be solved exactly as the Mk 1 Computer would solve it. Four hours were allowed to complete the exam. The MK 1 Computer was a dual purpose electro-mechanical machine capable of solving either a surface or an anti-aircraft fire control problems and generate gun orders and ballistic data for a 5 inch 38 caliber gun battery.

When not in the classroom, we instructors were busy overhauling various fire control equipment and installing said equipment on a two level concrete platform 400 feet long parallel to the beach. Thus, hands on experience was provided to the students in operation of various fire control equipment which included rangefinders, radars, computers, stable elements, gun directors, gyroscopic lead computing gun sights, and twin 40 mm gun mounts.

Later on, I was placed in charge of a visual-optical laboratory supervising four sailors in its operation. This lab had been established at the behest of our local National Defense Research Council, (NDRC), headed up by Dr. Imus, Ph.D. in psychology. It was necessary to process each student in the school through this lab. There were approximately seventeen hundred students at any one time in the school. The object being to evaluate each individual's ability to see stereoscopically, and to see that the results were placed in the respective students records. Fortunately this assignment ended after about four months. Dr. Imus and I did not get along too well.

One Saturday morning, I had arranged with the Executive Officer, for my men and myself to be excused from Captains Inspection while we evaluated results of a large number of students tested the day before. We were in the lab in the process of reducing the data when Dr. Imus entered and informed me that he had spoken to the Executive Officer and assured him that we could be finished in time to stand inspection. I blew my top. In no uncertain terms, I let him know he had no authority to interfere in military matters. After I called him everything but a preachers son, he looked at me and remarked, "Herriford, I simply do not understand what you are talking about".

After leaving the lab, I was placed in charge of installation and maintenance of Light Director Systems. This comprised 2 each Mark 52 systems, having Mark 14 lead computing gun sights. 1 Mark 63 system with a Mark 15 lead computing gun sight; and a Mark 57 experimental system having a 3 axis Rate Gyro Stabilizer, the Navy's first All-Electronic Fire Control Computer, plus a Ballistic Wind Computer. The Mark 57 system was a product of The Applied Physics Laboratory, John Hopkins University, Silver Spring, Maryland. It fell my lot to install, adjust, and place this system in operation. This project proved quite a task in that none of our people knew anything about it including myself. It took me thirty days to complete the installation and I learned the system in the process.

The last of May 1945, I took the exam for Chief Fire Controlman and was selected. I was elevated to Chief on the first of June and received orders to the Advanced Fire Control School in Washington, D.C. and had departed by 15 June. Ten days leave was granted in route, so I went to Tulsa to visit my mother, brothers and sisters. That was the last time I saw my brother Richard (Dick) Roy, as he was killed in a hunting accident the following November. He was fifteen years old.

15

Back to Advanced Fire Control School

As I was reporting in at the main gate of the Naval Receiving Station, Ana Costia, Washington, D.C. I observed Paul Otto Burch walking through the gate. There was a woman on his arm and like myself, he was wearing a CPO uniform. Jumping up, I ran out of the gate house and yelled "hey! P. Otto where do you think you are going?" He was most surprised to see me. We shook hands after which he introduced his wife, Marjorie to me. She was from Charleston, S.C. where Paul had been stationed for a period of time, the home port of his ship the USS Johnston, DD-557 being there. Burch and I went through boot camp at San Diego in the same Company 26 of 1940. We were both ordered to USS Detroit where we were shipmates until spring of 1943. Both of us became Fire Controlmen in the "F" Division. Which of us left Detroit first, I do not remember, but it had to be within a month of each other. Upon comparing notes we found both of us would be in the same class at the Advanced Fire Control School.

The CPO Quarters were in the Naval Gun Factory across the Anacostia River from the Receiving Station where the school was located. Summer was just coming on, this being the latter part of June, 1945. Air conditioning was relegated to open windows with fans and few of the latter. One did not sleep in those days in D.C. You sweltered in your bed until you died of exhaustion and perspiring until awakening

in the morning to find a wet outline of where you had laid on the bedding. Fortunately, there was a cleaning establishment directly across
from the S-E eleventh street gate. Sometimes a dress uniform could be
worn a second time without cleaning. Our cleaning bills were quite
high. We were permitted to wear wash uniforms to school. This, however, required a clean change every day to the extent our laundry bills
were also quite high.

The class size approximated 35 students, but this number was dou-
bled by conducting both day and night classes. For two weeks, one
would attend day classes then shift to night classes for two weeks. Over
on Eighth Street about two blocks up from the main gate of the Naval
Gun Factory was a gin mill known as The Farm House. All the bar
maids had been there for a long time and had become quite familiar
with various fire control equipments and nomenclature. Different
booths in the place had schematics etched in the table tops of various
systems. If a student failed to understand something in the schematic
just ask one of the bar maids and she would usually come up with the
right answer. It was rumored in the school that the Farm House was
part of the course.

Altogether, I spent perhaps 4 or 5 nights in the place. It simply did
not interest me. There was sawdust on the floor and everything in the
place appeared to have been thrown together. The women's head (Rest
Room) was situated in one rear corner of the main bar room and
looked as if it was an after thought. Anyway, the three-piece combo
played from a makeshift stage atop the ladies rest room. One night the
combo was so carried away with their playing all three fell through the
stage into the women's room. Fortunately, no one was using the ladies
room at the time, and to the best of my knowledge no one was hurt.

The course of instruction in the school was basically the 5 inch, 38
caliber dual purpose gun battery found in destroyers as well as cruisers,

battleships, and in some auxiliaries. Length of the course—33 weeks. Burch and I were in the same class.

About 20 weeks into the course, who appeared at the school but Lt. J.E. Stewar, our former Chief Fire Controlman from the USS Detroit. He was looking for people to staff his Fire Control Division aboard the newly commissioned aircraft carrier USS Midway, CV-41. Stewart said he was going immediately over to the Bureau of Naval Personnel, (BUPERS) and get both Paul and myself assigned to the Midway upon completion of school. He was no sooner out the door when first Burch followed by me appeared in the school Executive Officer's office with similar stories that went something like this, "women we were going with were pregnant and we felt the need to get out of town." While it was never disclosed to either of us, we felt that Stewart had talked to the Executive Officer about us prior his departure. In any case, the Exec expressed no objections to our termination and by 1600 that day; we each had orders to new destroyers under construction. Paul went to Charleston, S.C. and me to Seattle, Washington. A number of years later we would again become shipmates aboard the USS Norton Sound, AVM-1, Guided Missile Experimental Ship.

I was ordered to the USS Hollister, DD-788 which was under construction at Todd Pacific Shipyards on Harbor Island in Seattle. I arrived and reported for duty the early part of November 1945. She was due for commissioning the following April. I had been dating my wife-to-be, Jaretta Mae Jordon, for several months prior to my orders, who had a 7 year old daughter. She was living in Baltimore, Maryland and we were married there on the evening of October 4, 1945.

16

New Construction

My orders to the Hollister took me to Norfolk, Virginia, to pick up a draft of nucleus crew members. The result was that my new bride, step-daughter and I were forced to live in a small two room, cockroach infested apartment for two weeks awaiting make-up of the draft I was supposed to escort. When the Receiving Station finally endorsed my orders and sent me on my way toward Seattle the draft I was supposed to shepherd turned out to be a single Water Tender First Class, (WT/1/c) by the name of Arnold from Alabama. This one individual caused me more trouble than twenty men ordinarily would have.

The name of this man was Arnold. He was a heavy drinker and must have brought several bottles aboard the train in his luggage. The trip progressed with little or no trouble until after we left Chicago, but things changed drastically from that time on. The Porter in our Pull-man car was a very smart-ass South Chicago black man. Immediately he and this southern sailor in my charge got into a row. Arnold, about three sheets in the wind threatened to throw the porter off the train, and was big enough to do so. This situation persisted throughout the balance of the trip to Seattle. It required my continuous attention to hold that sailor in line. My new bride and I experienced our first fric-tion because so much of my time was required away from her trying to keep this sailor in check and away from the porter.

While in Norfolk it was my pleasure to visit the new aircraft carrier USS Midway, CV-41. She had just arrived at the Naval Station from

Newport News Shipbuilding and Dry Dock Company following her commissioning. I made it a point not to encounter the Fire Control Officer, Lt. J.E. Stewart, my former Chief Fire Controlman aboard USS Detroit. Frankly, I did not want anything to do with "Bird Farms". My forte was Gun **Fire Control** and in the black shoe navy, this had priority over everything else where I was concerned. On an aircraft carrier, the airplanes and their operations took top billing with gunnery coming in a poor second.

I explained my circumstances to the Chief Fire Control Man regarding Stewart. He gave me a cook's tour of the ship from one deck level below the hanger deck to the mark 37 Gun Directors in the island superstructure. Midway, when commissioned had 18, 5-inch 54 caliber dual purpose guns along with 84, 40mm and 28, 20mm antiaircraft guns. All these were subsequently removed.

The CPO Quarters in Midway were very far forward, one deck level below the hanger deck. It came to my attention that the Chief Fire Controlman would have to carry a lunch providing he planned to visit all units of his responsibility during a single day. That was one large ship. She was a beautiful ship but not for me.

We were two weeks in Norfolk, during which time I spent days at the Naval Receiving Station awaiting the make up of the Draft of men I was supposed to escort to Seattle. Jaretta and Shirley were more or less confined to that stinking little cockroach infested apartment during the day. Jaretta was one of the cleanest housekeepers it has ever been my privilege to know. Let me tell you, after two weeks that place was spotless and the cockroaches were almost nonexistent.

Early one evening, we put Shirley in a movie and went into a bar a couple doors down the street to have a beer or two and dance a little while waiting for the movie to end. Jaretta and I were sitting in a booth when all at once the owner behind the bar got into an argument with a big sailor. The owner took out a pistol from under the bar and threatened to shoot the sailor. Before realizing what I was doing, I found myself between the two trying to calm both down. I remember asking the owner to put the gun away and then persuaded the sailor to leave. Next thing I remember was sitting in the booth with Jaretta shaking like a leaf at the thought of what I had done.

We arrived in Seattle pretty well worn out. Investigation at COM 13, (Commandant 13th Naval District) revealed no military housing available, but we were referred to a Government housing office in Kirkland, across Lake Washington from Seattle. There we found a place to live, but it required me to ride four different buses plus a ferry boat across Lake Washington, for a distance of 17 miles that took 2 to 2 1/2 hours one way to Harbor Island where the USS Hollister, DD-788 was being built. To add to the problem, it was raining when we arrived in Seattle and this was the same weather we experienced for the next 29 days and nights. The sun never revealed itself during that entire period. Winter came on after that to make matters worse, with snow and cold weather.

While at the Fire Control School in Florida, I installed several "Light Director" systems. Upon my first visit to Todd Pacific Shipyards where the USS Yellowstone, AD-27 and USS James E. Kyes, DD-787 were under construction I was asked if I would like to work for the shipyard in a moonlighting status. My answer was yes, primarily because we were hard pressed for money and I could still look after my Pre-Commissioning duties. Little did I know at the time that some LtJg in the bureau of Supply and Accounts was sitting on my application for Family Allowance and would do so for the next 8 months despite the fact Navy was withholding $60.00 each month from my pay to cover my portion of Family Allowance. Believe me, we were becoming quite destitute when finally I wrote a letter as if written by Jaretta to Senator

David I. Walsh, chairman of the Senate Naval Affairs Committee stating our situation and plight.

Prior to this time, I had contacted Navy Relief Society, the Chaplain of Com 13, and everyone else I could think of trying to get a resolution to my problem to no avail. Within a week, we had a letter from Senator Walsh stating that he had been in contact with the Chief of the Navy Bureau of Supplies and Accounts, (BU S&A) and that we could expect resolution very shortly. Three days later, we received a letter of apology and a check for $800.00 from Chief of BU S&A.

I worked for Todd Pacific for six weeks when I received a telegram informing me my brother Richard (Dick) Roy had been killed in a hunting accident. I obtained 10 days leave and the Navy Relief Society loaned me $25.00 cash and purchased a round trip ticket for me to return to Oklahoma. Mind you, this was over Thanksgiving that I would be gone. Leaving the $25.00 with Jaretta and Shirley and with approximately $5.00 cash in my pocket, I departed. On the return trip, my train became stranded in western Wyoming. By now I was flat broke and had missed a couple meals, when a soldier loaned me a dollar to get something to eat. Wouldn't you know when I got home I discovered a one dollar bill with Hawaii stamped on it tucked away in my wallet.

Upon my return to duty, I did not return to work for Todd Pacific, but devoted all my time to activities related to commissioning the Hollister. Still, we were quartered at the Naval Quarters on Harbor Island separate from the shipyard. There were watches and various other duties to be performed by four watch sections. A watch list was published each day containing names and times. On a Thursday afternoon just prior to posting of the watch list, I departed about 10 minutes prior to liberty call. My watch section did not have the duty until Friday. However, the CO of the naval facility took it upon himself to change my watch section to Thursday just prior to posting the watch list, thus putting me in the present duty section. There was a chief torpedoman that I believe informed the CO I had departed early, which brought about the change in the watch list. This chief was in the Hollister Pre-Commissioning Detail. Other Chiefs informed me he had better not commission the ship if he knew what was good for him, and he did not.

When I arrived at the barracks on Friday morning, I was immediately summoned to the CO's office by the Chief Master of Arms who remained outside the CO's open office door after I entered. The CO began calling me every kind of demeaning name he could think of, then informed me he was charging me with jumping ship and failing to stand an assigned watch. The latter part of his statement was news to me since I had not been on the watch list at the time of my departure the afternoon before. I was placed under arrest and sent to Pier 92, the Receiving Station in Seattle in the escort of two Chief Petty Officers.

Upon arrival there the Brig Officer, a Navy Lieutenant, after reading the orders for confinement turned to me and remarked, "Chief, what kind of a son-of-a-bitch have you got over there that would send a CPO over here to be confined on such minor charge? He then told me he could not put me in the brig, but that I would have to remain on the base over the weekend. Upon finding out about foul names, the CO had called me. The Brig Officer informed me I could bring charges for redress of wrong, providing I could come up with a witness to the event. The Chief Master of Arms who had been standing outside the open doorway denied hearing anything, thus ending this event by dropping all charges against me.

The USS Hollister, DD-788 was commissioned on 22 April 1946 at Todd Pacific Shipyards on Harbor Island, Seattle Washington. The ship within a very few days departed for six weeks of Underway Training in San Diego, California. My wife, Jaretta skimped and saved for

several weeks to obtain a pair of ladies hose for the commissioning ceremony, which were still in very short supply. However, on that eventful
day it rained and she was very embarrassed that the rain had spotted her
hose with their cheap dye job.

I shipped over for another six years on the first of April. When the
ship returned to Seattle I was granted 30 days leave. I purchased a used
car and we packed up our things and moved to San Diego in July 1946
where Hollister was to be home-ported following her post shakedown
yard period.

Upon my return to duty, the manpower shortage became very critical. The normal compliment of Fire Controlmen for this class ship was
18. Instead, beside myself I had a second class PO and a third class PO
with no strikers until the Executive Officer placed two men at my dis-
posal, one of which I could select for a striker. We were required to
keep all equipment in operation. In our four-ship division, it became
necessary to pool the crews to have manpower to operate two of the
ships one week with auxiliary crews manning the two ships remaining
at the mooring buoy, then switching over to the other two ships the following week. Firing practices were being conducted nearly every time
we went to sea, preparing for our deployment to the Far East in
November, 1946. Often as not, my Gunnery Officer would fail to
inform me of a gunnery practice until after we had gone to general
quarters. On several occasions, my Third Class P.O. alerted me to the
fact we were going to shoot. It was my responsibility to compute the
Initial Velocity setting and enter it into the computer just prior to a
shoot. About ten minutes were required for this operation. Often I
would have to delay opening fire in order to accomplish this task for
lack of input information regarding magazine temperatures, air density,
type of ammunition, wind direction and velocity, along with several

other factors. The manpower situation was so drastic that some Chief Petty Officers were standing OOD watches while underway.

17

Deployed to China

Early in November 1946, our Destroyer division was making plans for departure to the Far East via Pearl Harbor and Guam. However, the Squadron Leader, USS James E. Kyes, DD-787 was without a Chief Fire Controlman for one reason or another. Anyway, guess who was delegated to fill that vacancy. Yours truly reported aboard the Kyes from the Hollister two or three days before our departure for the Orient.

Jaretta, my wife, along with our daughter Shirley, (eight years old) and I, had been making plans for a month or six weeks for this event. We knew our date for leaving the States and I was so concerned about leaving them that we decided they, Jaretta and Shirley would return to Marion, Indiana, and live with her relatives while I was overseas in WESTPAC. During the latter 1940's, and this was November of 1946 the duration of overseas deployment was nine months.

Liberty expired at midnight preceding the day of our departure. Therefore, Jaretta and Shirley came down to the fleet landing at the foot of Broadway in San Diego to see me off in the last boat to leave the landing at the appointed hour. That proved to be a mistake I vowed never to make again. It was a very heart-wrenching experience for all three of us, saying good-bye. Be assured, thereafter our good-byes were said at home.

Fortunately, I was well acquainted with most of the Officers and Chief Petty Officers on the Kyes, so I immediately fit right in. It was understood we would be involved with occupation duties following so closely upon the end of WW-II once we arrived in the Far East. This assumption proved to be correct, but many of us counted on being permitted to wear working uniform most of the time, except for when on watch or going ashore. Boy, was that ever a mistake. The ship had no sooner cleared the outer channel buoy than the Commodore had the word passed that "uniform of the day" for all Officers and Chief Petty Officers was service dress blue. I had brought only one service dress blue uniform along. By the time we got to Shanghai, where I managed to get it cleaned, that suit of blues would stand on its own.

There were four Destroyers in our Division cruising together until we departed Guam, after which we split up with the Hollister and Kyes, setting a course for Shanghai while the other two headed for Hong Kong. On the way, we stopped off in Pearl Harbor for about a week to conduct some gunnery exercises and again when we reached Guam, we were in port for four or five days to refuel and take on provisions. After leaving Guam the Hollister and Kyes conducted, a long range offset gunnery exercise using live service ammunition in our six 5" guns.

Prior to going to General Quarters, I went down to the plotting room and set a 100 mil right deflection spot into the Mark 1A Fire Control Computer and locked it in. You see, the firing ship was to use the other ship as a target, but with the 100 mil right deflection spot applied, the fall of shot should occur 600 yards astern and over the wake of the target ship at a range of 6 thousand yards. Unfortunately, my Follow-up Operator on the computer released the spring-loaded spot knob after we went to General Quarters, thus removing the 100-mil right offset spot.

A rake party was set up on the fantail of the Hollister to score our firing from the Kyes. Upon receiving the command from our skipper to commence firing, I fired the first six-gun salvo and just following the second salvo I heard some commotion over the TBS radio speaker and recognized something was amiss. Without receiving a command from the skipper, I immediately reached over my head, actuated the cease firing claxon and gave the command to cease-fire. Even before looking, I knew what had happened to my computer setup. I made sure the Follow-up Operator had reset the 100 mil right deflection spot then reported the situation to the Captain, where upon he ordered a resumption of firing. Later the skipper chided me by asking if I had a grudge with those people on the Hollister. After we arrived in Shanghai several of the Hollister CPO's told me the first salvo was directly over their wake about 300 yards astern with 6 detonations and that the second salvo was approximately 200 yards astern smack over their wake with 6 detonations. About that time, all exposed people on Hollister were seeking shelter. Suffice it to say, the balance of the gunnery exercise concluded with no further excitement, other than both ships had a good shoot.

We entered the Yangtze and steamed up river some twenty or thirty miles to the Wangpu River, which we then took to Shanghai. That was a scary experience. I recall an LST, apparently sold to China, coming down river almost head on. The river current was in the neighborhood of 8 knots and that coupled with approximately 8 knots of LST speed was something to behold. We passed with something like 20 yards between us having a differential speed of 24 knots. Our two ships tied up to separate mooring buoys in the middle of the Wangpu about a quarter mile off Custom Jetty in the International Settlement. This was my first trip to Shanghai, and from out in the middle of the river, it was evident the city was filthy.

Wouldn't you know, it was my luck to have Shore Patrol the first day and night in Shanghai. I was Chief in Charge of eight sailors to report to the Permanent Shore Patrol at police headquarters. Knowing absolutely nothing about Shanghai was bad enough, but not being able to speak the language made it extremely difficult. I was directed to take my eight Shore Patrolmen to a very busy intersection in the International Settlement with instructions to keep all military personnel from going toward the Wangpu jail where a riot was being staged by a crowd of communist university students.

As it turned out the assigned intersection was one large mass of pedestrians. There must have been ten thousand people with not a single motor vehicle in sight. The pedestrians gathered around us Navy personnel just staring at us, so tightly we could hardly move. It took me thirty minutes to station two Shore Patrolmen on each of the four corners. However, there was a traffic control officer on a podium in the middle of the intersection doing a sort of dance ritual and going through the motions of directing traffic as if there were many motor vehicles present. I later learned that these police were graded and rated on their dance routines.

One night, Chief Gunners Mate Brown and I were returning from the Navy Club out on Bubbling Well Road at Nanking Road, beyond the Race Course. Each of us were in separate rickshaws, when all of a sudden Brown's coolie swung into an alley while my Coolie kept going toward Custom Jetty. Try as I did, I could not get my coolie to follow the other rickshaw. Upon arriving at the dock, I reported the incident to the Shore Patrol, but before they could take any action, another rickshaw arrived with Brown. He had not been harmed, but they relieved him of all his valuables, and then turned him over to the lowliest coolie present to take him to the Jetty.

The wildest ride I have ever had occurred in Shanghai on the way back to the Police Station from our Shore Patrol activity. We were in a Chinese Nationalist Army vehicle with a soldier at the wheel, siren going and red lights flashing. The driver would approach the rear of a stopped streetcar, whip out around the streetcar disregarding the presence of passengers entering or exiting and zip right through their midst. How no one was struck is a miracle to me. I can still see wide eyed Chinese with mouths wide open at the shock of nearly being run down.

We left Shanghai about mid December, our destination being Hong Kong. On the way, however, we replenished our provisions and took on fuel from a sea train out in the East China Sea. In order to obtain one case of Irish potatoes it was necessary to take one case of carrots and one case of turnips or two cases of one or the other. Believe me, I have eaten carrots prepared every way you can imagine. The flour provided was what they called Truman Flour unbleached and loaded with weevils. For the first few weeks, we could pick them out, but after that they became so bad that we simply quit eating bread.

Regarding the flour loaded with weevils, the University of Minnesota published a paper extolling the nutritional value of weevils and emphasizing there was no detriment to human health.

We spent Christmas, 1946, and New Years 1947 in Hong Kong. I wired a dozen red roses to Jaretta from there for Christmas. Later when I returned home, she gave me a fit for my extravagance. During this time, another CPO and I were strolling around the city on Victoria Island when we came upon an elderly Chinese gentleman standing in the yard of what was apparently his residence. He spoke to us in English and we became involved in conversation that lasted for fifteen or twenty minutes. As it turned out, he was the owner of the company that produced Tiger Balm products, some of which were quite popular in the U.S.

Shortly after New Year 1947, the Kyes was ordered to Tsingtao, China situated on the south shore of a peninsula extending out into the Yellow Sea about 400 miles southeast of Beijing. We were moored to a wharf about half a mile from the U.S. Navy hospital ship USS Comfort. Our purpose for being there was to support a contingent of marines stationed in the vicinity. From time to time, we could hear firing of field artillery in the hills, related to encounters between the Chinese Nationalists and Chinese Communists. While in Tsingtao, I obtained permission from my skipper to see if the hospital ship would remove my tonsils. At the time, it was thought we would be in port for at least two weeks. All arrangements for the operation were completed and I was being checked in on the hospital ship when my skipper called, stating I must be back aboard Kyes within a week or otherwise send me back. I was sent back. Would you believe that in twenty-one years of naval service, I tried any number of times to have my tonsils removed, but in every instance, I contracted an infection and the medics would not touch them. I was retired from the Navy over two years before I finally got rid of them. Doctor Sammy Lee, the 1934 Olympic Diving Champion performed the operation in 1962.

From Tsingtao, we went to Pusan, Korea where we patrolled the coast for about a month, intercepting gun runners from North Korea. After that we went to Sasebo, Japan thence to Kagoshima and Nagasaki. It was in Kagoshima where I met Paul Revere from Boston Massachusetts. He was a Captain in the Army commanding a MAG, (Military Army Government) unit.

We were at sea on our way to Yokosuka, Japan, when I received orders to the Advanced Fire Control School in Washington, D.C. This particular evening another CPO and I went up to the Radio Shack where we found the Chief Radioman with a set of ear phones on, one ear piece connected to a receiver from which he was copying press reports and the other ear piece connected to another receiver from which he was copying Navy communications. All the while we were talking to this individual he was typing on two separate typewriters respective of the receivers he was monitoring.

When we first entered the Radio Shack the Chief Radioman, asked me if I had seen my orders. Thinking he was just making conversation, I replied in the negative and we continued talking. Finally, after about ten minutes he brought up the subject of my orders again and pointed to a clipboard hanging on an equipment rack. Suffice it to say I was surprised beyond belief when I read the dispatch. It was orders for me to go to the advanced Fire Control School in Washington, D.C.

I was detached from Kyes soon after arriving in Yokosuka and reported to CPO Quarters in the navy yard. There I met another Chief Fire Controlman whose name I believe was Rex, also with orders to school. For about three nights, we boozed it up at the CPO Club prior to our flight out of Honida Airport near Tokyo. During one evening at the CPO Club when I was about "Three Sheets in the Wind" I remarked to Rex that while in the Advanced Fire Control School, I intended to take the entrance exam for the Fire Control Technician School and upon completion of that school was going into Guided Missiles.

That night, under the influence of a few drinks, I was expressing my utmost desires for my career, while realizing at the same time the remoteness of such ever happening. However, would you believe that is exactly the course my naval career took. More on that later.

Just prior to my departure from Kyes, I was given 10 inoculations, 5 in each arm. When I checked in at Hanida Airport, an Army Medic requested to see my shot record. Unfortunately, I could not produce it since I had packed it in my luggage, which by this time was already loaded on the airplane. Lo and behold, I was given 9 more shots before being permitted to depart.

Our airplane was a Navy R5D (a DC-4), a four-engine propeller job bound for Guam with a load of freight. Bucket seats along each side facing inboard accommodated about 10 passengers. We left Japan shortly after dark and encountered a violent storm within 30 minutes of our departure. All lights were off in the cabin, but lightening managed to keep the interior pretty well illuminated. Several times there was the sensation of an express elevator in a tall building dropping out from under us. The Plane Captain informed us that we were encountering down drafts that in several instances dropped us as much as a thousand feet. I recall looking out the window in the direction we were heading, after leaving the storm and seeing lights on Guam well in excess of a hundred miles before we arrived. We arrived about 0200 local time, the flight having approximated eight hours in duration.

We passengers were quartered in an abandoned barracks near the airfield, equipped with nothing but double deck bunks with no mattresses, just bare springs. It was as if we had been forgotten until about noon when a bus picked us up, took us to a mess hall, then to the airfield where we boarded another four-engine airplane. This time however, it was a plush aircraft operated by Naval Air Transport Service, (NATS). They fed us hot meals every four hours in flight with Waves as flight attendants. The flight landed at Johnson Island and I'll swear the wheels touched the water when we landed and that the starboard wheel was in the water as we turned around at the end of the runway. The flight time from Guam to Honolulu was in the neighborhood of 18 hours. There was a three day layover at Pearl Harbor until the next scheduled flight to the States. The last leg turned out to be a Marine flight, also plush R5D to Moffet Field. All flights into Moffet were required to make an instrument landing, which we did, then took off again, circled around and made a regular landing. The flight time from Honolulu to San Francisco in those days was 12 hours in propeller powered airplanes. The Navy R5D airplane was the equivalent of the DC4 flown by the airlines in those days.

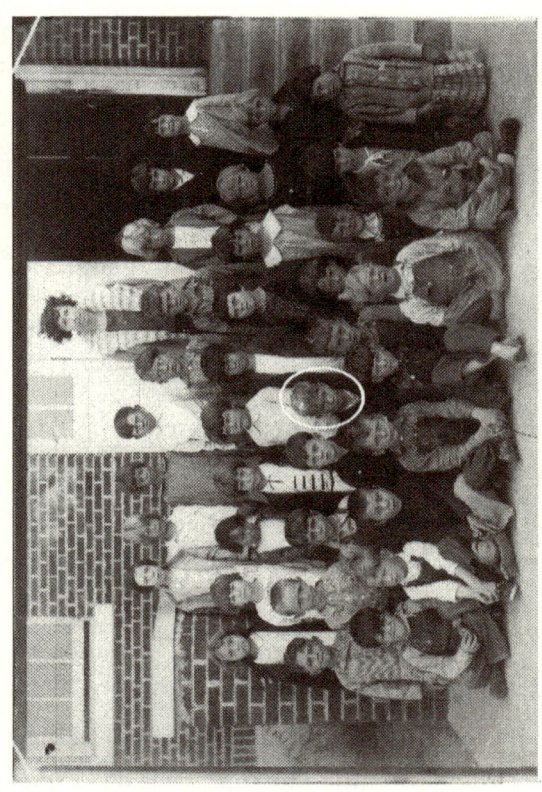

School, October, 1928

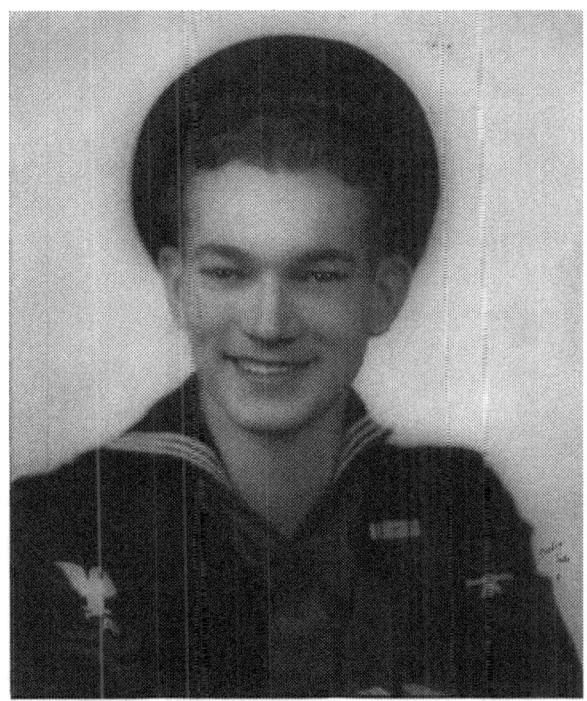

1942

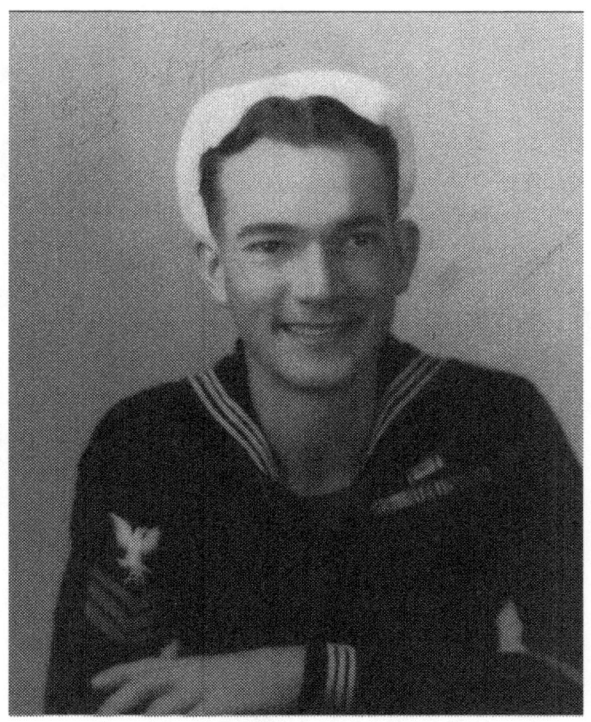

1944

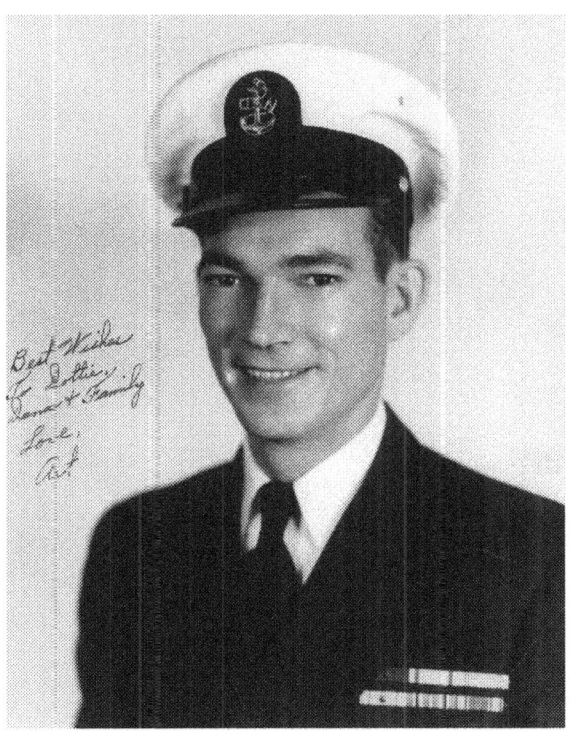

November, 1957

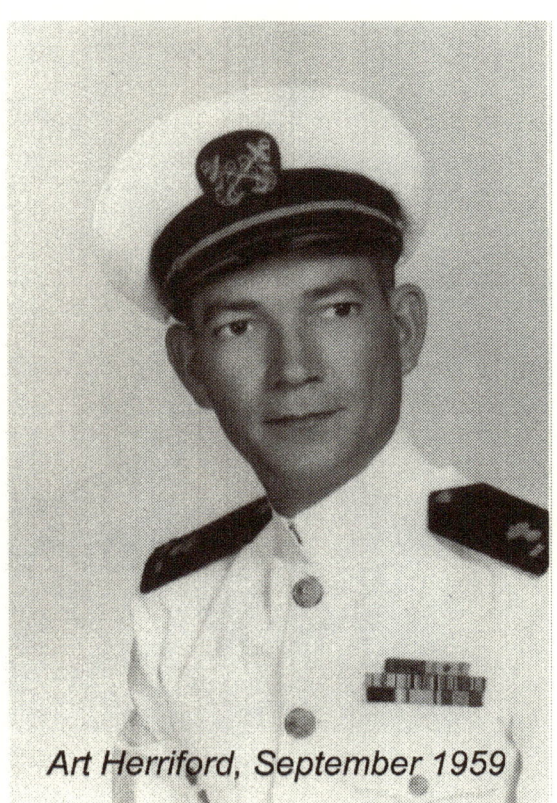

Art Herriford, September 1959

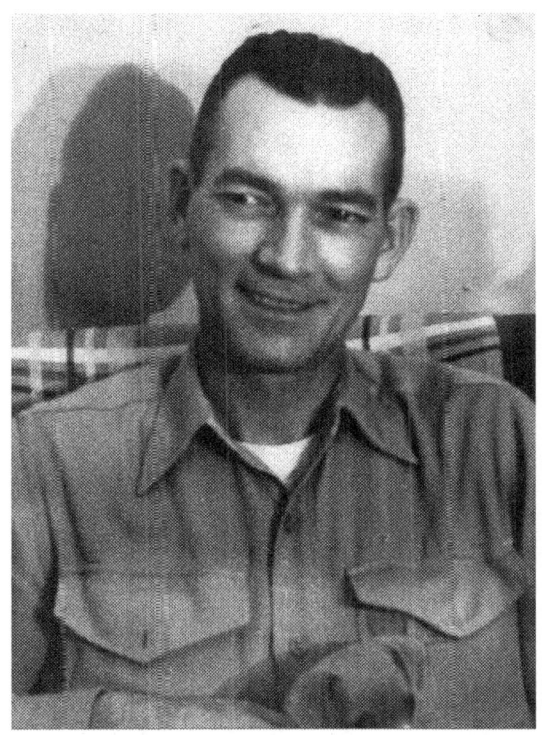

1967

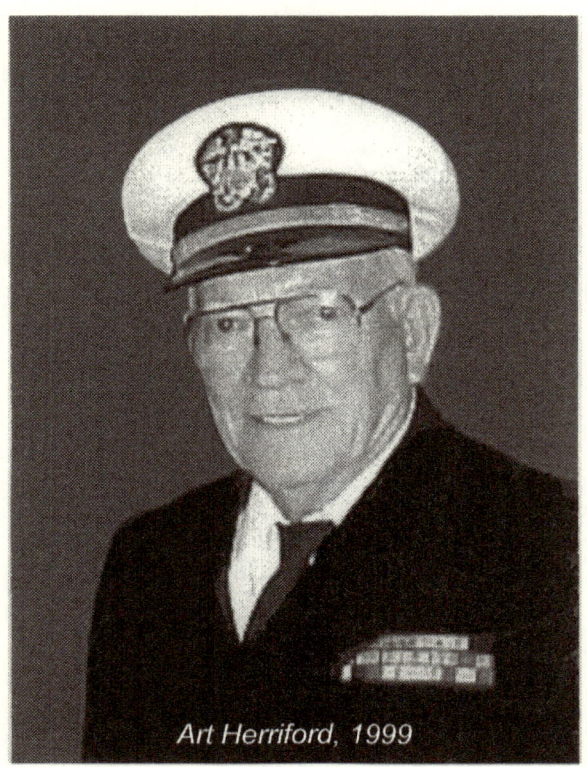

Art Herriford, 1999

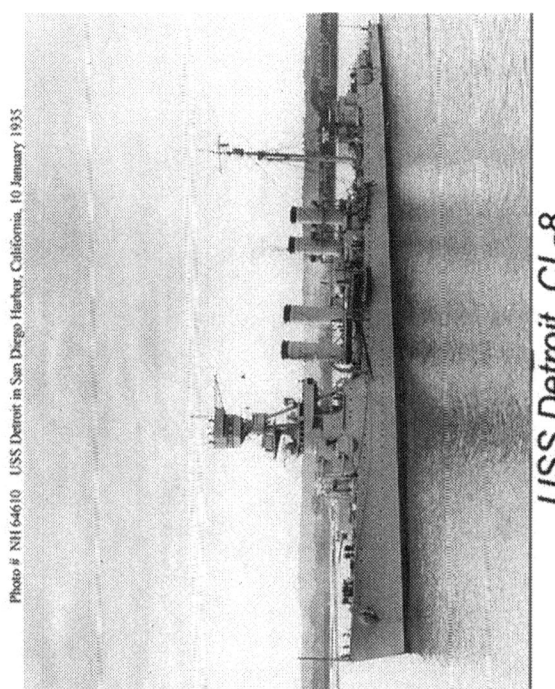

Photo # NH 64610 USS Detroit in San Diego Harbor, California, 10 January 1935

USS Detroit, CL-8

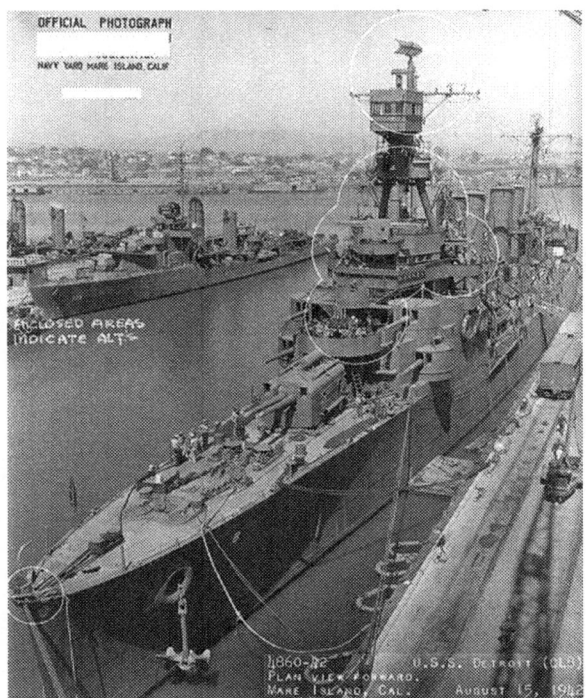

Light Cruiser, USS Detroit, CL-8

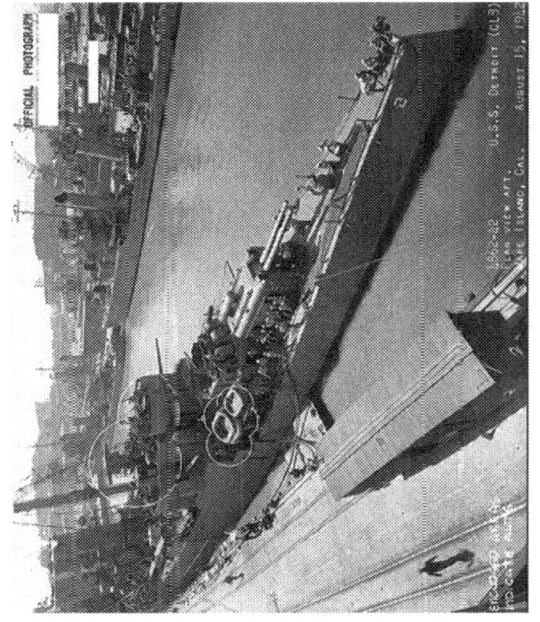

Stern of USS Detroit, CL-8 in Mare Island Navy Yard

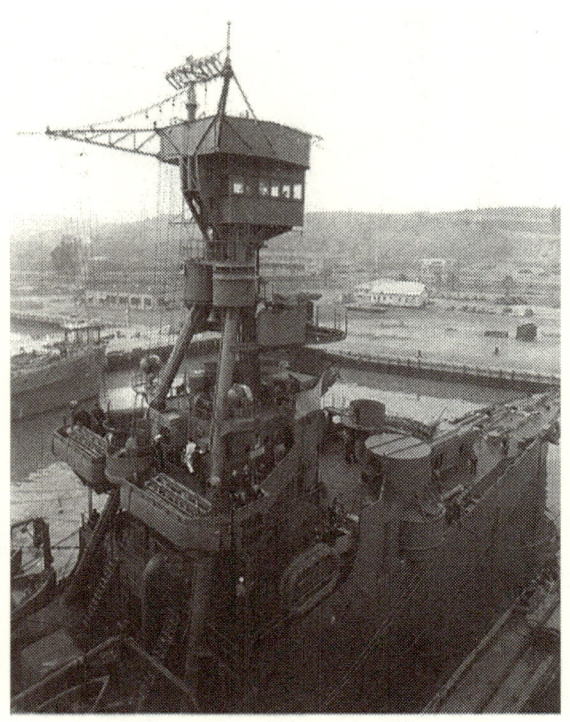

Forward Superstructure USS Detroit, CL-8

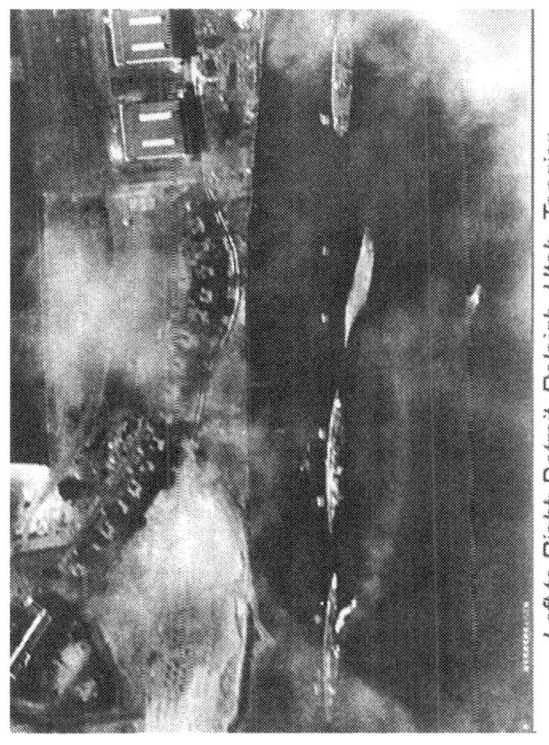

Left to Right: Detroit, Raleigh, Utah, Tangier

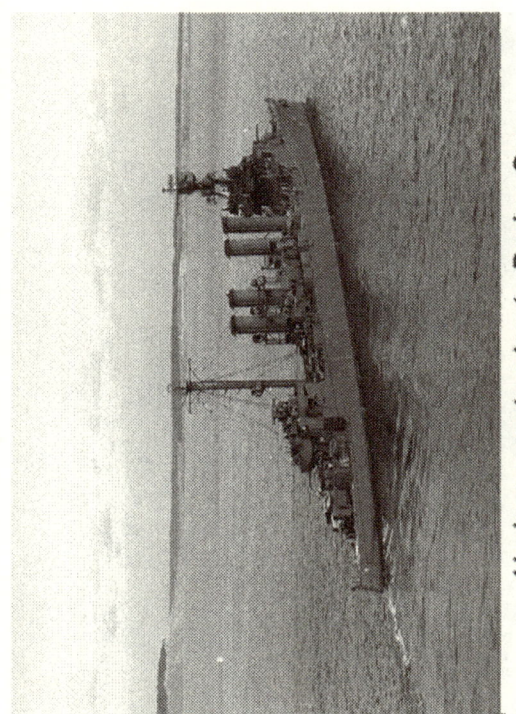

Underway returning to Bering Sea and Aleutian Islands

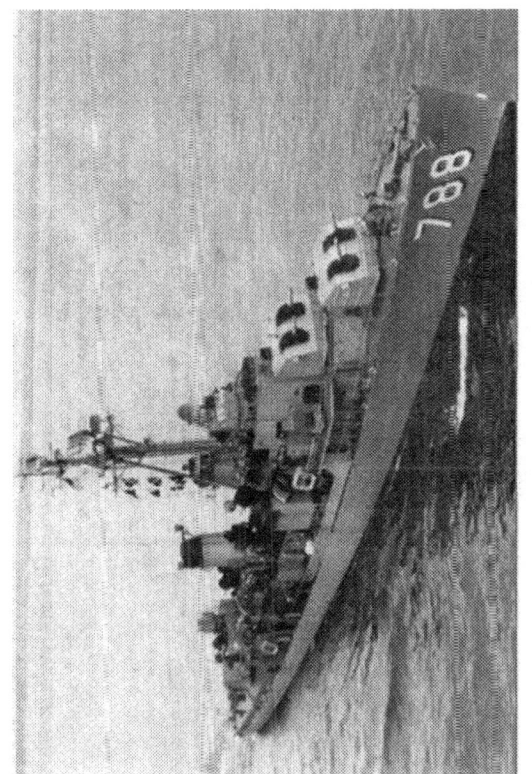

USS Hollister, Destroyer

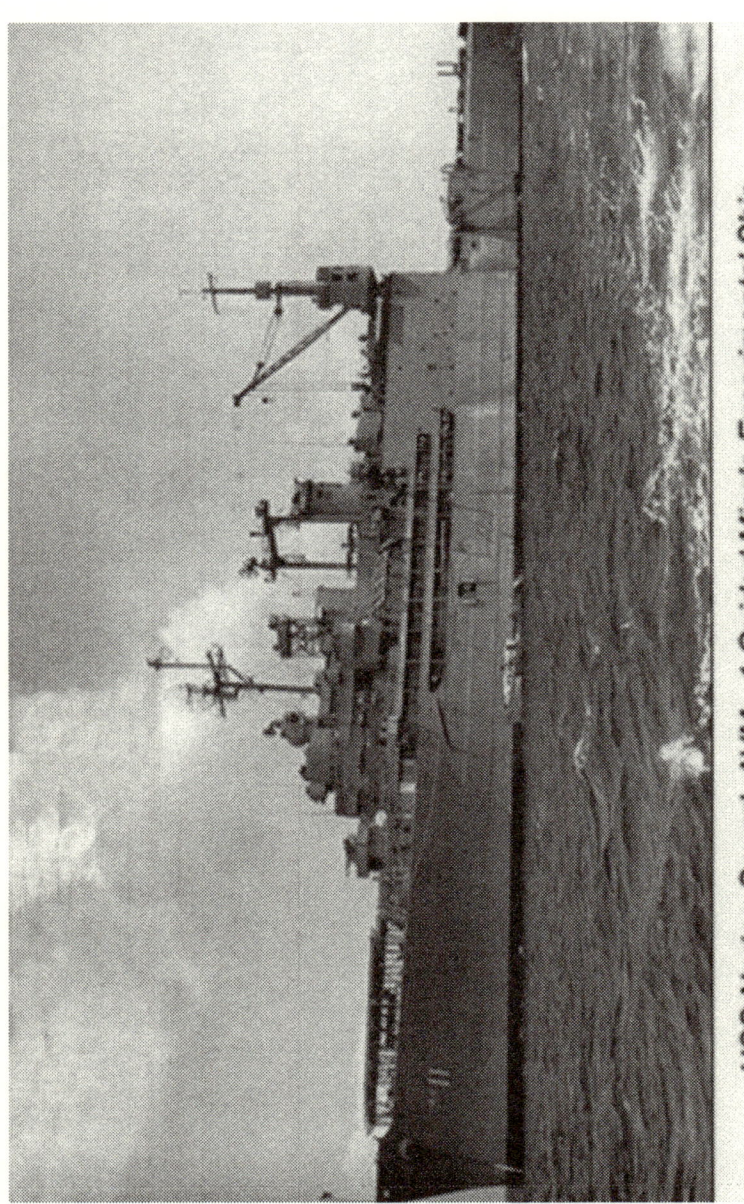

USS Norton Sound, AVM - 1 Guided Missle Experimental Ship

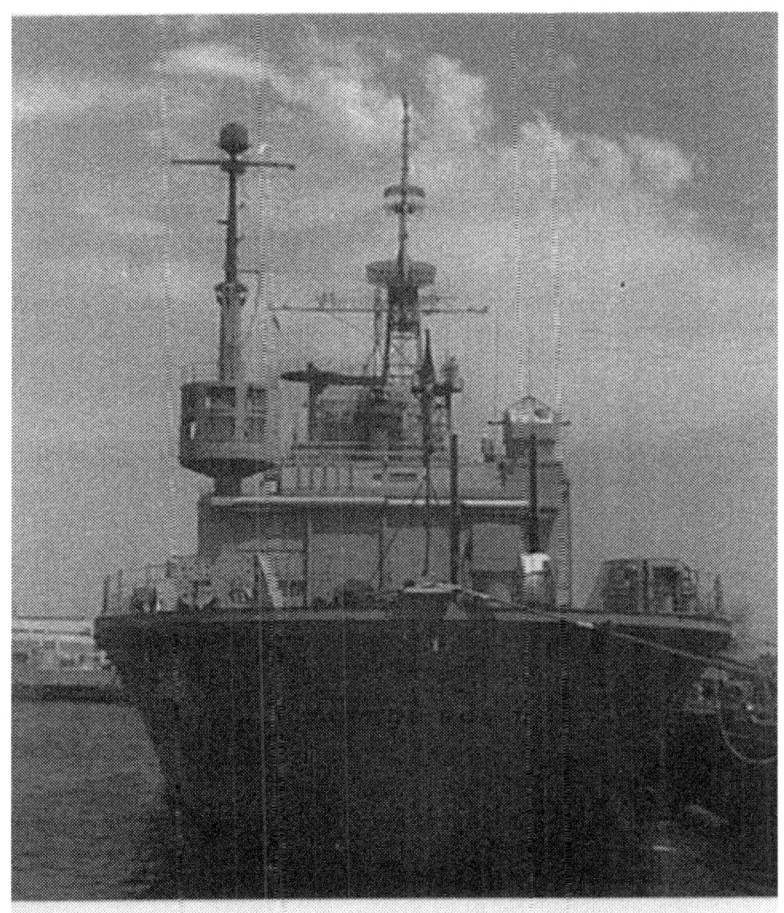

Stern view USS Norton Sound

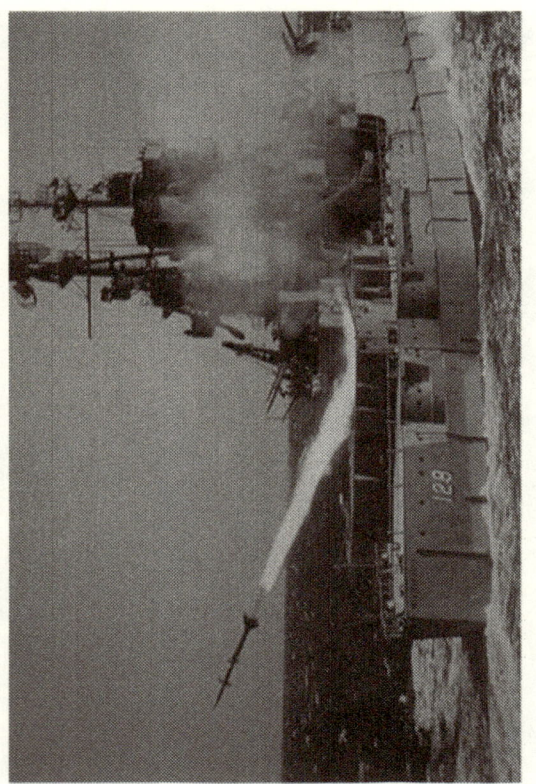

Launching Terrier Missile from USS Mississippi, EAG-128

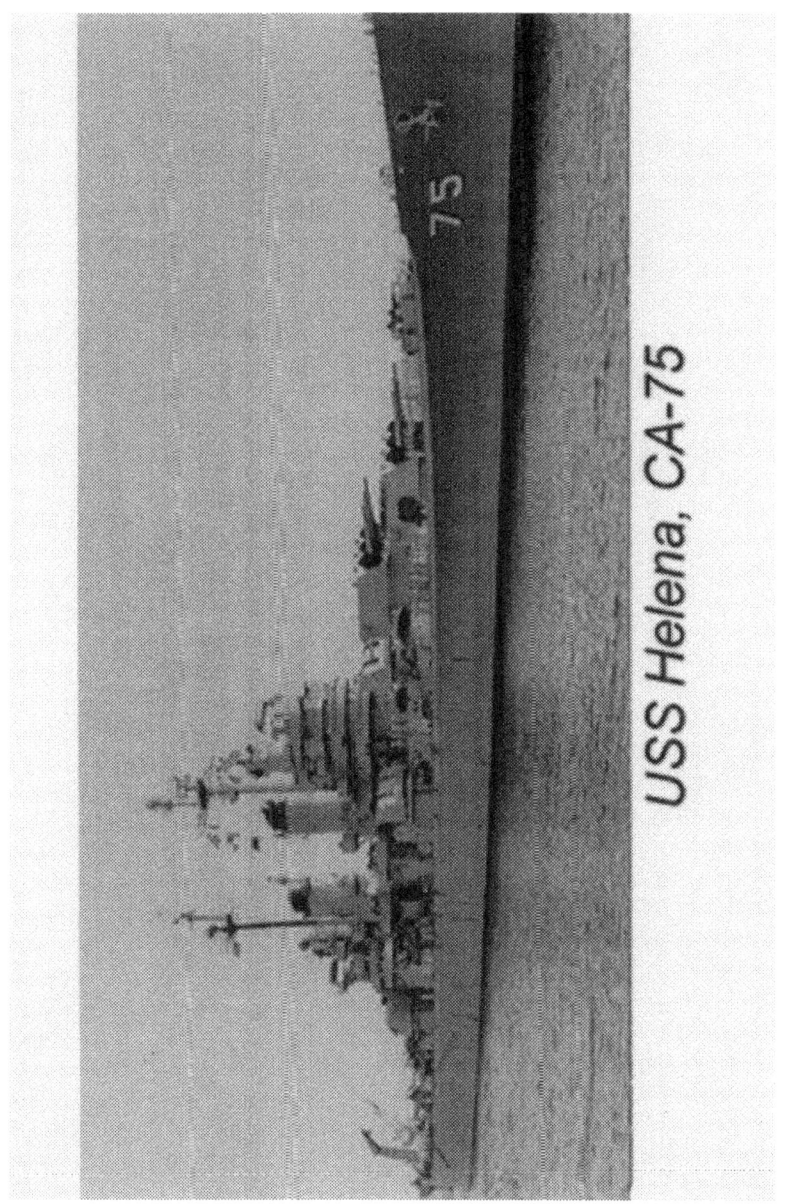

USS Helena, CA-75

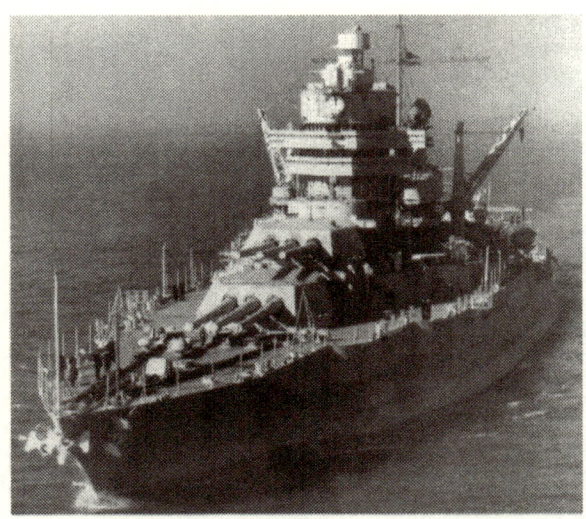

Battleship USS Mississippi
prior to conversion to
experimental ship

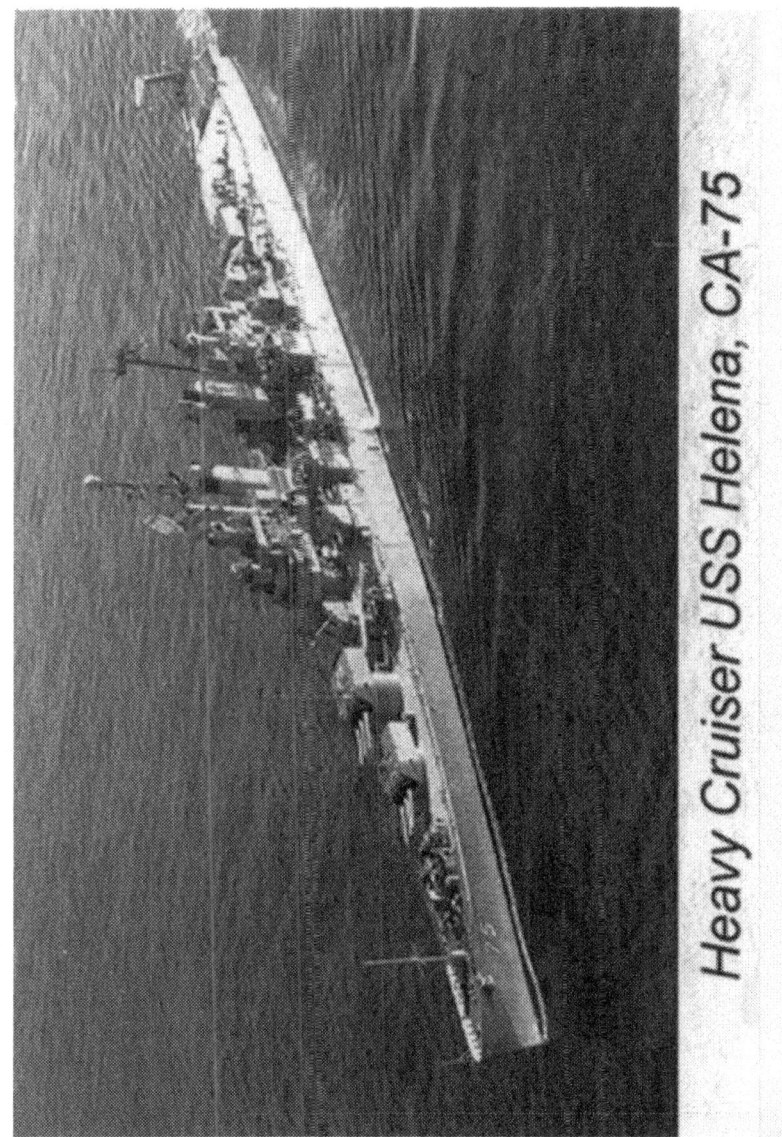

Heavy Cruiser USS Helena, CA-75

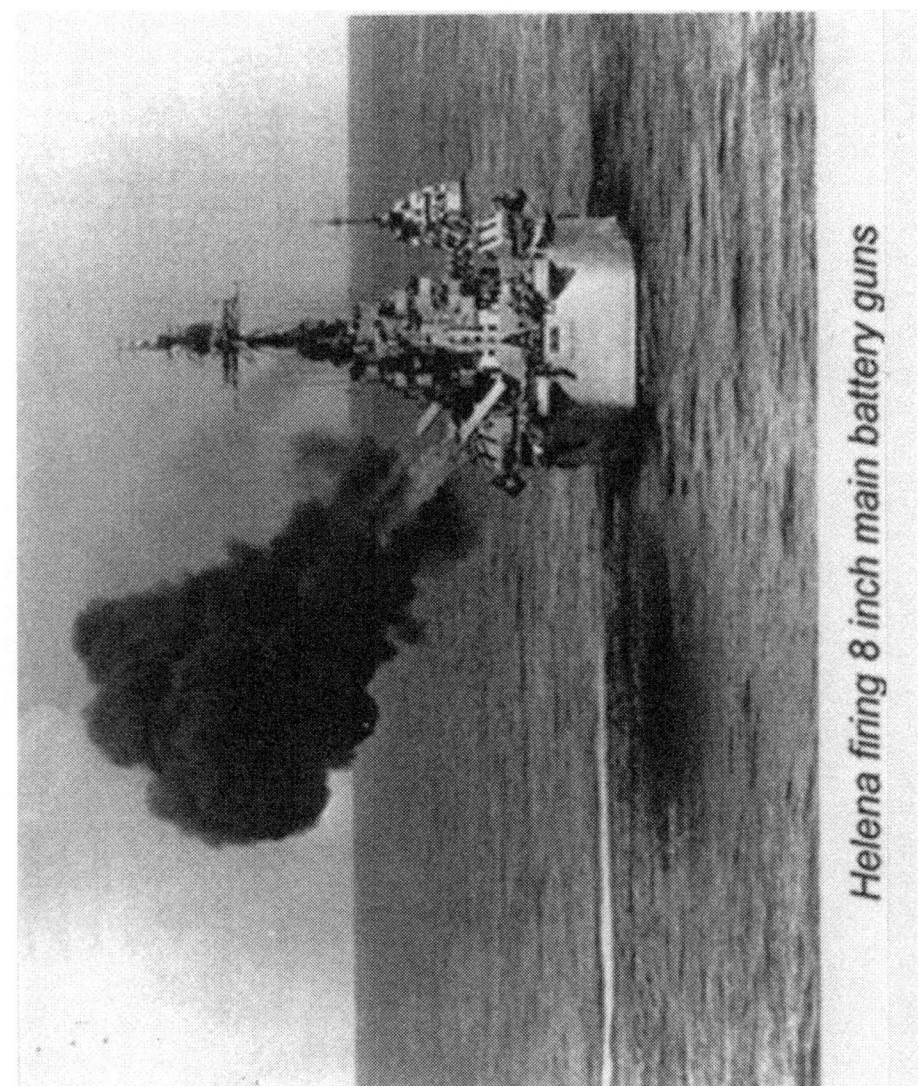

Helena firing 8 inch main battery guns

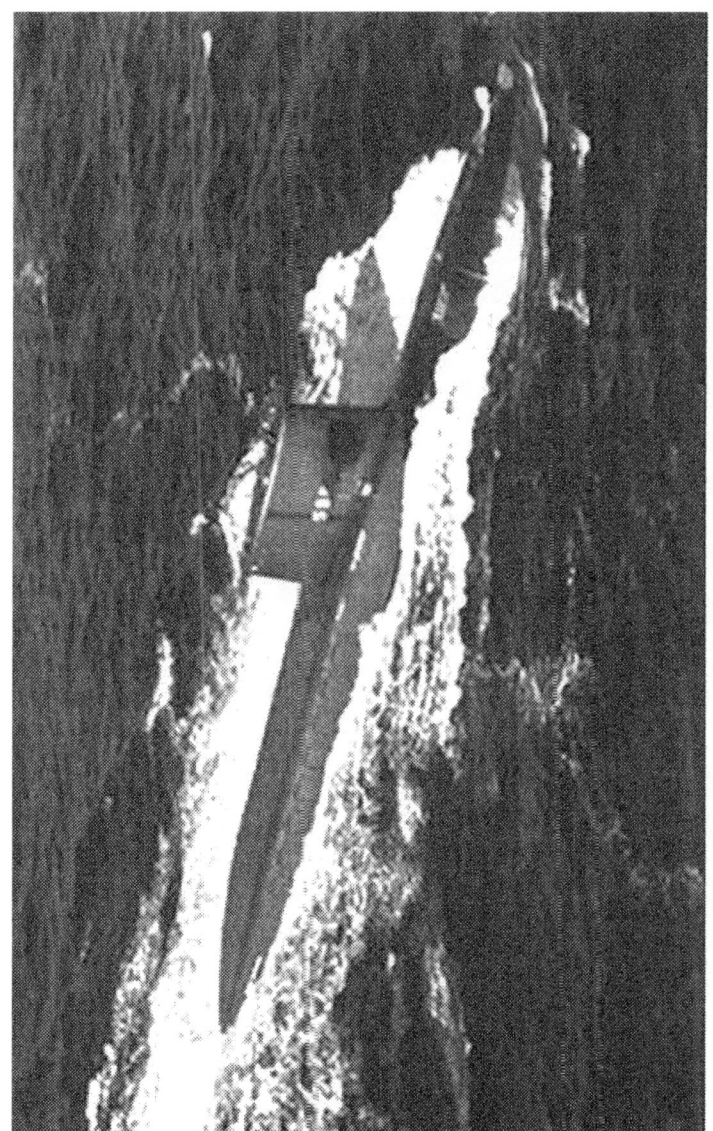

First Polaris Submarine SSBN-598

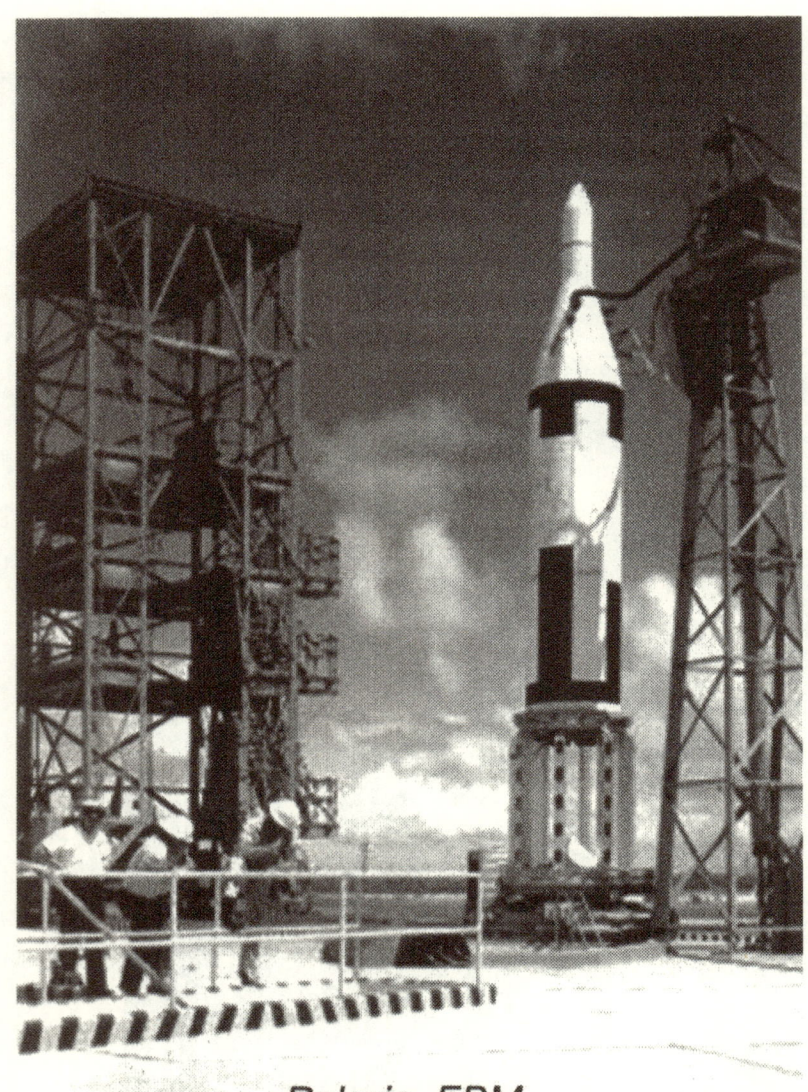

Polaris, FBM

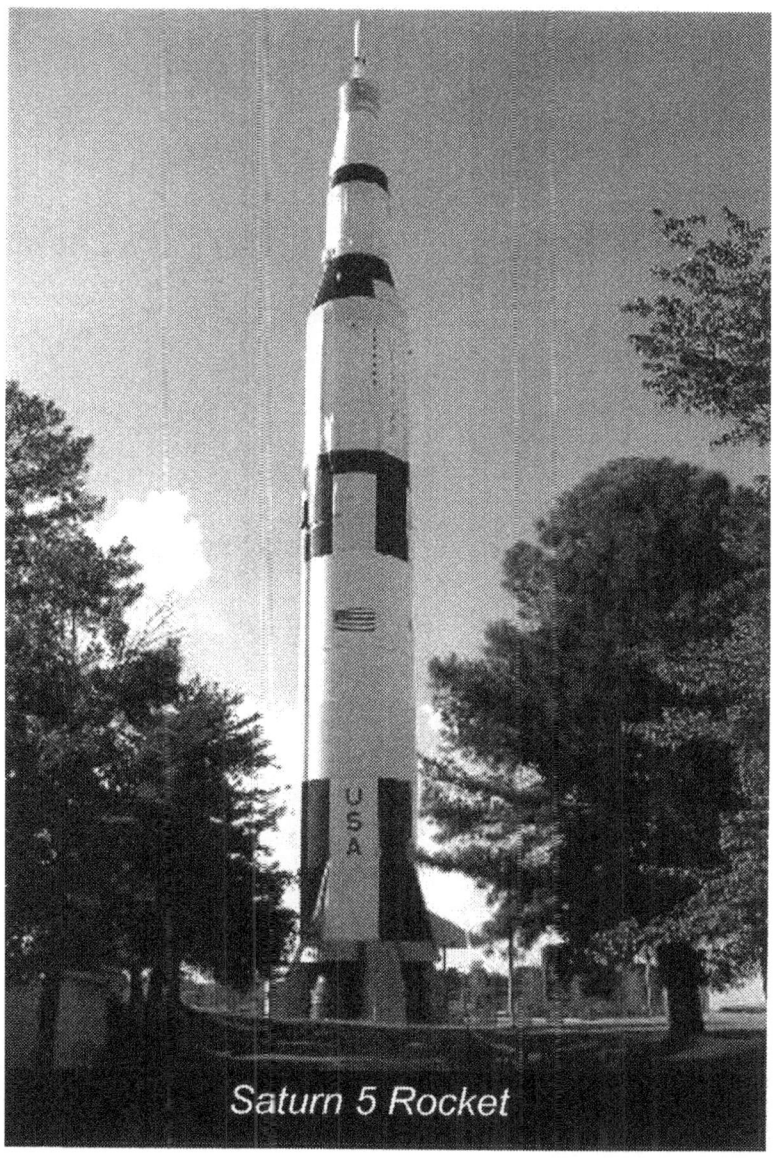

Saturn 5 Rocket

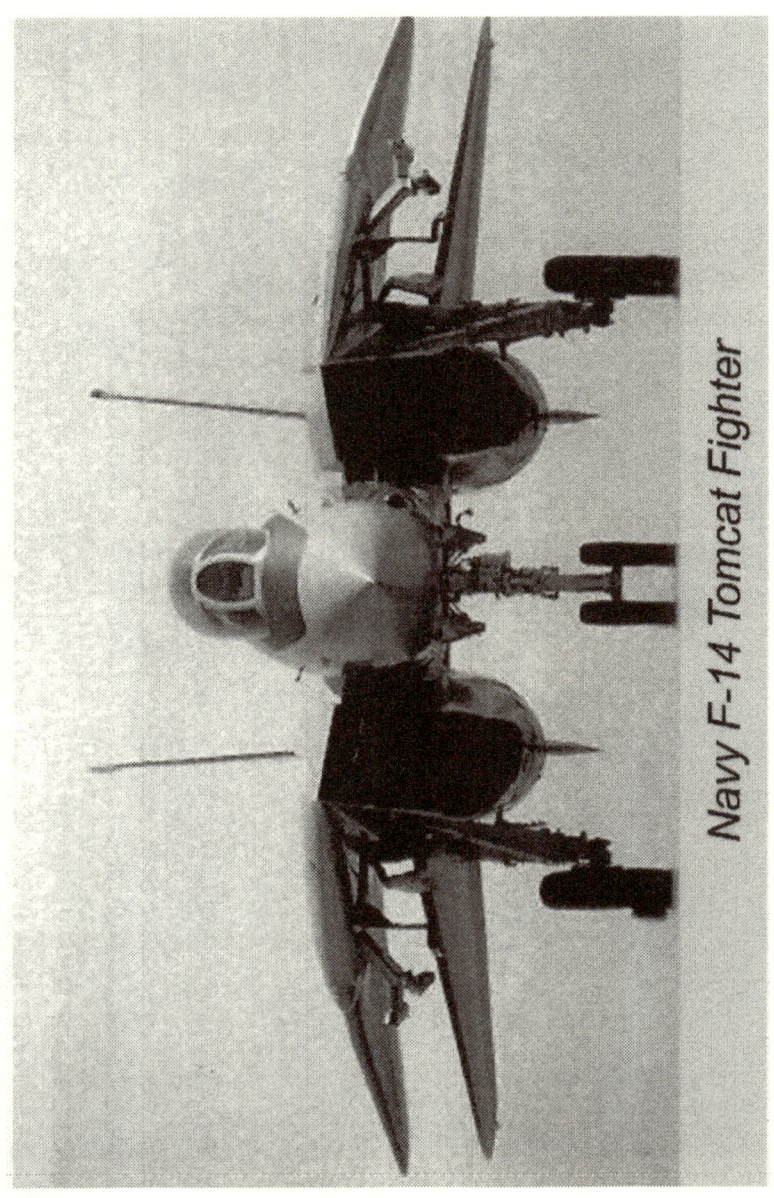

Navy F-14 Tomcat Fighter

18

Fire Control Technician School

I was authorized about 20 days leave before reporting to school. Taking a train to Marion, Indiana from San Francisco, it was necessary to change trains in Chicago. I was most anxious to see my wife and daughter and had to this point never met Jaretta's parents. There were about 15 or 20 other relatives present. Right off the bat I committed a grave mistake when I mistook Jaretta's Aunt Clara for her mother. However, I soon was acquainted with them all. This was about a week before my 24th birthday on 17 April 1947.

Jaretta and I decided to purchase a car, recognizing it would be a necessity once we got back to Washington, D.C. Automobiles were still very hard to come by so soon after the war. A waiting period of 6 months to a year was necessary for buying a new car and good used cars were quite scarce also. However, with strings pulled by Jaretta's Uncle Frank, we found a nice little 1937 Ford that seemed to be in good condition and capable of getting us to Washington. It proved to be quite reliable, except both heads on it's 60 horse power V8 engine were warped. About every two or three months I would have to replace the head gaskets. I got pretty proficient at that job.

To find a place to live around Washington in those days was all but impossible. We settled for a bedroom with kitchen privileges out in West Lanham Hills, Maryland about 10 or 12 miles from the advanced Fire Control School situated in Anacostia, D.C. The course of instruction in the Advanced Fire Control School at that time was 33 weeks long. Would you know one of the staff officers at the school was an old shipmate of mine on the USS Detroit. His name was Larry Moore, but somewhere along the line someone hung the nickname of "Sugar" on him. When I last knew him, he was a Fire Controlman 1/c. Furthermore, both he and Rex, the Chief I returned to the States with from Japan, were also old shipmates. As it turned out, Rex reported into the school several weeks ahead of me.

Not many people liked Moore because he was known as a user of people. He once bragged he would rather wear gold in this man's Navy than have friends. To my knowledge, he had few if any friends.

While still in Japan, having learned that we had a mutual acquaintance in Moore, I confided to Rex a number of my dislikes of Moore. By the time I reported to the school Rex had spilled his guts to Lt. Moore. This I was not aware of until it came time for me to take the entrance exam for the Fire Control Technician School. Lo and behold, who was to administer the exam to me but Lt. Moore. It took 1-1/2 days to take this exam, so Moore and I sequestered ourselves for nearly two days in an empty class room. Early on, Moore let me know that Rex had spilled his guts. Figuring that my chances for getting into the Fire Control Technician School were all but gone, I proceeded to tell Moore what I thought of him. One must have been in the top 10% of those taking the exam to be admitted to the school. To my surprise, I was in that top 10% and entered the Technician School two weeks after completing the Advanced School.

Jaretta went to work at Wilber Rogers, a chic ladies apparel shop in the heart of Washington not far from the White House. She became the top sales lady in that establishment. Her income was sorely needed at that time. Normally she would ride the bus to work and I would wait around after school to pick her up from work.

After almost 7 months of living in West Lanham Hills, we were fortunate enough to have found a 25 foot house trailer for sale, and bought it from a retired Army Colonel for $1400.00 at 6% simple interest. It was like a mansion to us. Although small, it was every thing we needed at that time. We located in a trailer park 7 miles south of Alexandria, Virginia, about a 12 mile drive to school.

The course of instruction in the Fire Control Technician School was 50 weeks until my class came along. At that time, a 6 week Fire Control Radar course was added. John Craven another old shipmate from days on the USS Detroit, was the instructor, having just completed the Electronic Technician school at Great Lakes Naval Training Center. Class size in Technician School was 10 to 12 students, whereas in the Advanced School, 36 students was common. I must tell you when in the Technician School as a Chief Petty Officer, I became "Captain of the Head". For those of you who are not familiar with naval terminology, I was responsible for cleaning the rest room. Our class sizes were quite small and made up of Chiefs and First Class Petty Officers. The student body therefore was responsible for cleanliness of the school facilities.

Normally, two weeks before graduation orders for further assignment were handed the class with those having seniority getting first choice. It so happened for my class no orders were received until after we had taken the final exam on Friday morning. Having completed the exam, we were instructed to go to the cafeteria and remain there until summoned. We were called back to the classroom about 11:45 when the orders were handed to us. The reason for the holdup was that three of us, myself included, were being ordered into a Guided Missile Program at the Applied Physics Laboratory, Johns Hopkins University, Silver Spring, Maryland.

The delay resulted from lack of completion of secret security clearances for the three of us. All other people in the class wanted to kill the three of us for the delay of orders, since they were deprived of lead time in preparing for transfer. As for myself, I also was extremely concerned regarding transfer orders up to this time. My house trailer needed tires and it had been impossible to save any money for travel. On several occasions, I had expressed my concern to the owner of the trailer court, where I was moonlighting as the court electrician. In every instance, he told me not to worry that I was not going anyplace. Each time it was my thought that he was just trying to sooth my anxiety. Little did I know that he had been interviewed on more than one occasion about me with regards to security clearance. The result of it all was that I did not have to move for several more months.

My new duty station located in Silver Spring, Maryland, required a drive of about 20 miles from where I was living; 7-miles south of Alexandria, Virginia across the District of Columbia into Maryland. Depending on time of day and traffic conditions, the average driving time approximated one hour.

This was on the job training. We were assigned to assist top scientists and engineers in new conceptual ideas and innovations. These people imparted knowledge to us that was far ahead of the times. For instance, I was initially assigned to assist Dr. Wilks, PHD in Physics who was investigating the principles of optics when incorporated in beams of Radio Frequency Emergency. In a lab setup, a 5-inch reading glass was inserted in the output beam of an X-band transmitter and the power meter on the receiver jumped up by a factor of 9 db. The same effect was observed when the reading glass was placed in front of the receiver input waveguide horn. Subsequently, a metallic lens antenna was designed that focused an RF beam from a scanner on the backside to a beam 1 degree in diameter on the front or target side when radiated through the metallic lens antenna. The Mark 25, Mod 6, Mod 6A, and Mod 7 Missile Guidance Radars utilized this antenna which was 7 ½ feet in diameter.

19

Guided Missile Research and Development

I reported to the Applied Physics Lab (APL) in Silver Spring, Maryland, just outside the District of Columbia, on Monday following graduation from Fire Control Technician School the previous Friday in the month of April 1949. The exact dates are not important. Two officers and fourteen enlisted personnel had been selected for "On The Job Training" under tutelage of various scientists and engineers in the process of developing several different guided missiles in the Navy's "Bumble Bee Program". We Navy people were formed up in a unit designated Guided Missile Training Unit 21, (GMTU-21). LCdr Arthur G. Hamilton USN was officer in charge of the unit and the only officer present when I reported for duty. I was a Chief Firecontrol Technician (CFT) and of the fourteen enlisted people assigned to this unit all were Chief Petty Officers, except three of my men, two of which were in my class in the Fire Control Technician School.

My class in the Fire Control Tech School was the first to receive instruction in Fire Control Radar Mark 25 Mod 2 . Having gained this information, I was assigned as **Crew Chief** with three other navy personnel to pursue development of a Missile Guidance Radar. The radar group at APL were already working to modify an Army model SCR-584 radar. We began by helping various engineers machine and develop a variety of waveguide and RF components for this unit. A little later I was assigned to work with Dr. Wilks who was investigating and applying the principal of optics to antenna systems for concentrating radar RF beams into known beam widths.

Dr. Wilks gave several lectures and demonstrations on his work. With a small high frequency (X-Band) RF transmitter set up on one side of the room and a compatible receiver on the other side, he would insert a 5 inch diameter magnifying glass into the transmitted RF beam, first at the transmitter then again at the receiver. A large galvanometer/ power meter mounted on the receiver indicated considerable gain in received signal strength in both instances. Following the lecture, Dr. Wilks would then proceed to prove mathematically to everyone present that what they had witnessed was impossible. However, sometime later he discovered the error in his computations, which did indeed make it possible.

My crew of three sailors and I were ordered to take a new type radar antenna to the Naval Research Laboratory where we spent three weeks assisting Lab people in measuring antenna gain, RF beam width and side lobes. This antenna was a 7 foot diameter **Metallic Lens** having an "A" frame to support a scanner on the rear side. Radio frequency, (RF) energy was radiated through the lens out into space. It so happened this was the antenna to be incorporated into the Navy's first missile guidance radar.

GMTU-21 was scheduled to deploy in March 1950 to China Lake, the Naval Ordnance Test Station, (NOTS) located in the most northern valley of the Mojave desert at Inyokern, California. I am in possession of a 2-1/2 hour video tape depicting the history of NOTS titled "The Secret City". However, in late September 1949, one of my people, Whittington, ET1/c and I were ordered on three months temporary additional duty to Reeves Instrument Corp. in New York City. Reeves landed the contract to modify a Mark 25, Mod 2 Fire Control

Radar to a Mod 6 Missile Guidance Radar. We were to receive instruction in this equipment and provide consultation to Reeves technical staff as needed. As it turned out, it fell my lot to have to write the system alignment and integration procedures for the technical manuals. The subsistence allowance was $5.00 a day for us naval personnel. We took a room at the YMCA and if it had not been for the various Reeves engineers taking us to lunch every day we would have starved to death.

Our orders for the first 3 months expired the first week in December. Whittington and I had heard we were to be extended for another 3 months, so we checked out before orders extending our stay arrived, and boarded a train for Washington. I caught hell from the officer in charge of the Guided Missile Training Unit along with several high placed civilians in the Navy Bureau of Ordnance. Anyway, they let us remain in Washington for a week and then sent us back to Reeves Instrument Corp. in N.Y. where we remained until 14 February 1950. Jaretta and I spent the most lonesome Christmas and New Year you can imagine in our 25 foot house trailer at Jerico,Long Island, N.Y. We had left Shirley, our daughter, with John and Maggie Craven in Washington. Maggie was expecting their first baby about that time.

We were so broke that I was cashing $25.00 savings bonds in order to put gasoline in the car to get to and from the Reeves Plant at Roosevelt Field. When I checked out at the Receiving Station in Brooklyn on the afternoon of Valentines Day, the CPO in the Pay Office informed me I was over paid by about $163.00 and that I had no money coming. I explained that I was being transferred to the Naval Ordnance Test Station at China Lake, California and that I was flat broke. There upon, he pretended not to have received the order to dock my pay and advanced travel expenses to me. We left Long Island just ahead of an ice storm bound for Washington, D.C. and from there a 10 day trip to China Lake, California, towing our 25 foot house trailer.

20

New York to California

It was after dark when we finally left Jerico, L.I. and it had begun to rain. All was going fine until we got near Trenton, N.J. about 11:00 p.m. when a rim on the trailer split and the tire blew. We managed to get into a trailer court for the night. However, I spent nearly all the next day running all over New Jersey trying to find a Graham wheel. This house trailer, 25 feet long, was built on a single axle and the **Graham** wheels were drop center, not commercial. Anyway, I found a wheel late in the day and got it mounted. We stayed over until the following morning before again pointing toward Washington. This wheel situation would come back to haunt me later in the trip to California.

After arriving at our old trailer court 7 miles south of Alexandria, Virginia, we stayed over one day then headed west taking the southern route along US 80. At 45 miles an hour it took 10 days to make the trip. We lost another trailer tire 15 miles east of Lordsburg, N.M. about 11:00PM on a high crowned two lane road with deep bar ditches on either side. While I had set emergency reflectors and flares the big 18 wheelers hardly slowed down. The Graham wheels had lug bolts, not studs and nuts as is now standard. Using a socket and breaker bar with a pipe extender/cheater, I could not loosen the lug bolts. Rather the hex bolt head simply rounded off on all 6 bolts. I worked until about 2:00AM using a hammer and chisel trying to get those bolts loose which had frozen in the hub. Finally, I became so tired that we climbed into the trailer and went to bed despite all the traffic on the road.

Next morning, a Sunday, I was able to remove the wheel, put it in the car and drive into Lordsburg. With a lot of luck, I was able to get the Goodyear dealer to open his store and make the tire replacement prior to his going to church. The failed tire which was purchased in Washington, D.C. when last there, had developed a bubble on the side wall and worn through against the wheel-well. There was no charge for the new tire, so after obtaining several new lug bolts, I returned to the trailer, mounted the wheel and we were on our way again.

Upon passing through Tucson, Arizona, we noticed a sign in front of a welding shop for rebuilding wheels from drop center to commercial. Well, would you know about 20 miles west of Tucson another rim split. Fortunately we were near a trailer court and we got into it. I blocked the trailer up, removed both wheels, and took them back to the welder where we had seen the sign. He agreed to rebuild them both for $25.00. Said they would be ready next morning. The following morning when I picked up the wheels, I learned the guy had worked all night rebuilding them.

Jaretta, Shirley and I were again on our way and never again experienced any trailer wheel problems. I was pulling the trailer with a 1948 Pontiac, 2-door sedan with a 6 cylinder engine and a Hydramatic transmission. Never had one bit of trouble with the car the entire trip. However, I began to wonder when we started up Cajon pass. It heated up a bit, so about half way up we stopped and had lunch. Remember this was in early March, 1950. There was no such thing as freeways in those days. Afterward, we proceeded over the pass and headed across the desert toward Inyokern on US 395. The further north we went the more desolate things became. The question in our minds was what possibly were we getting into? About mid-afternoon, we arrived in Inyokern and took a spot in the Inyokern Hotel Trailer Court. Other members of Guided Missile Training Unit 21 were already there.

The Naval Ordnance Test Station, (NOTS) was 9 miles East at China Lake. While there was a trailer park on the base, it was full. Therefore, those of us located in Inyokern were destined to remain there for the time being. My work required a 15 mile drive one way, 9 miles to the Base then another 6 miles down into the dry lake bottom where we were installing a guided missile R & D launch site. Finally, after about two months, those of us living in trailers were allowed to move into the old Trailer Court in the old initial section of the Base, which had more or less been abandoned.

NOTS was considered to be a remote area, and indeed it was. As such, it was necessary for the Navy to provide both housing and shopping facilities for approximately ten thousand civil service and professional people on the base. At this time, Ridgecrest was not much more than a cross road, although it was growing. Los Angeles was about 150 miles south and slightly west while Bakersfield was about 130 miles almost due west over the south end of the high Sierra Nevada Mountains. NOTS, China Lake was located in Indian Wells Valley, the northern most pocket of the Mojave Desert. With the facilities provided by the Navy there was little or no reason for anyone to leave the area, unless on personal business.

A large butler building had been installed to be our Weapons Control Center at the edge of the alkali deposits in the dry lake bed on what was known as G-1 Range. Adjacent to that about 30 feet away a concrete pad was poured, upon which, a 16 ton Mark 37 Gun Director was installed, and that in turn was the mount upon which the Missile Guidance Radar was installed. A twin rail launcher was located about 50 feet away from the Director/Radar assembly, separated by a berm about 15 feet high and covered with asphalt to serve as a blast deflector.

Later, during missile launches, I had much appreciation for that dike because it became my job to give a running commentary over the PA system of the missile attitude and responses during the first few thousand yards of flight. My head and shoulders were exposed above the Director shield and the blast from the fourteen hundred pounds of propellant in the booster rocket would almost tear my head off. Besides that, large chunks of asphalt rained down on me. Sometime before this, I escorted a party of dignitaries over to G-2 Range, a half mile away, to witness firing of a booster rocket from each launcher arm for test. At that distance, the blast report had people with ringing ears and shaking their heads. The booster exceeded **mach-1** in less than 9 inches of travel; therefore, the shock wave added to the blast of the rocket motor.

Inside the Weapons Control Center, we located an Electro-Mechanical Computer controlling a graphic plotter, a modified Destroyer Fire Control Switchboard, about eight cabinets of Missile Guidance Radar electronics, various other instrumentation and the Weapons Control Station.

A team of ordnance people from the Naval Gun Factory in Washington,D.C. came out to NOTS to make the installation of this Missile Launch Site. When they arrived, an agreement was reached whereby I would assign one of my men to each of theirs. We thus performed half the installation under their supervision, and at the same time we learned the system inside out. I engineered the necessary changes to the Fire Control Switchboard to accommodate it to missile functions. There are about 50 large 8-position rotary switches having as many as 12 pancakes on some switches on this unit.

The modification effort on this switchboard knocked me out of possibly being selected to a commission as Limited Duty Officer, (LDO). It happened that the number three officer in seniority in Guided Missile Unit-21 was at the moment working in the Range Design Section of Michaelson Laboratory. While I was responsible for system integration at the launch site, this officer started marking up various drawings of the switchboard, then sending them out to me to be approved. After about six or seven iterations of my rejecting his red-lined drawings, he gave in and told me to accomplish the task, but to keep very accurate records so that Range Design could at some later date commit the changes to releasable drawings. This I did, and when the job was complete, I had a ruled sheet of paper showing the electrical changes to each cable for each switch in the switchboard totaling about 10 to 15 pages in approximately 30 different manila envelopes.

I was working at a drafting table in the rear of a trailer behind the Weapons Control Center. This was also the headquarters for the ordnance gang from the Naval Gun Factory. The officer mentioned above came into the trailer and commenced bragging to the ordnance gang about how he had redesigned the Switchboard. Like a damned fool, I exploded and told the Lt. off in front of everyone. They all knew that I had actually engineered the job. Suffice it to say I did not make LDO.

Upon completion of the Launch Site, personnel of the Guided Missile Unit were responsible for manning and operating all equipment during missile shoots. In those days guided missiles were all more or less hand constructed with telemetry instrumentation installed on every facet. The countdown for launch commenced at minus 24 hours. This made for some mighty long days on the range. After about the third or fourth shoot, we were able to shrink the time and let people go home for a few hours rest. Before the first shoot however, after completion of installation, Cmdr Bud Slack, Officer in Charge, GMTU#21 scheduled us to man the system at 04:00AM for the purpose of debugging and proof-of-station. Two of us arrived at 2 minutes after 04:00. Cmdr. Slack looked at the clock and remarked "Gentlemen, when I say 04:00 by God I mean 4:00". After that, everything went smoothly.

One Sunday a group of us GMTU people with our families was permitted to take several jeeps from the base motor pool for an outing up on Wild Horse Mesa on the north end of the military reservation. Our women folk packed lunches and we set out. Louisiana Butte, in the Volcano Range was at the north end of China Dry Lake, 13 miles north of our launch site. We visited petroglyphs in a canyon at the base of the mountain, "Louisiana Butte", and then drove up over one side of the butte to the mesa. There we met Old Pop. He was an old prospector the Navy had hired, made him a US Marshal and stationed him on the north end of the reservation to keep out interlopers. Old Pop showed us all over the mesa. We saw wild burros, wild horses and explored the entire area, driving where neither roads nor trails existed. That was quite an outing.

GMTU-21 was due to transfer to the USS Norton Sound, AVM-1, home ported in Port Hueneme, California in December 1950. This was a Guided Missile Experimental ship, formerly a Large Seaplane Tender. Several of us from the unit paid a one day visit to the ship in late summer 1950 in company of Cmdr Slack for the purpose of becoming acquainted. In preparation for this move Ray and Helen Kuhlow, along with Jaretta and I bought new homes in Reseda, California. Reseda is located about the center of San Fernando Valley. Several others either bought or rented in the same general area, with the idea of car-pooling to Port Hueneme, a distance of 50 miles.

When we departed NOTS I turned the Missile Guidance Radar over to a Civil Service technician who was rated as being sharp in this field. Two years later I was to find out how inept he was. More on this subject later.

21

Commander Gay

We left NOTS and moved into our new home in the San Fernando Valley the mid part of December 1950, after which I reported aboard the USS Norton Sound for duty. Our car pool got off to a good start since several of us in the Guided missile unit had purchased in the neighborhood. It was generally an hour's drive from Reseda to Port Hueneme, California. Mind you, this was before Freeway/Interstate highways.

The Norton Sound occupied a permanent berth there with special mooring lines designed to hold the ship within 6 inches of lateral movement in any direction. This requirement resulted from having to radiate our Missile Guidance Radar into an RF waveguide receiving horn on a shore tower at head of the pier.

My radar crew spent 16 to 18 hours a day radiating that tower. Various groups of engineers from Convair in San Diego, GE or some other outfit were authorized 54 hours per week for which they got paid overtime for all over 40 hours. These people would approach me with the idea of working 11 or 12 hours a day until they completed their effort and would then be out of my hair. Initially that sounded fine, except that when the first group was finished there was another group waiting to do the same thing. Once these people got their overtime hours in, usually about mid afternoon on Friday, they would insist that my radar Scanner had failed. Thus, they would pack their bags and head home for the weekend, while my men and I would spend the weekend overhauling the Scanner. It took several weeks for us to catch on to their scheme and at which time Cmdr. Slack put a stop to it. However, in the meantime, my crew had become walking zombies. Suffice it to say, this put a kink in my participating in the car pool. Often as not, I found myself working overtime without benefit of any compensation. I do believe I have worked many 26 hour days in succession while in the naval service.

On days we were scheduled to fire a missile, the ship would get underway about 0900. We would steam out onto the Pacific Missile Range off Point Mugu about 50 miles, conduct the shoot, steam back into port and usually be tied up by 1600, (4:00PM). Not bad duty, except we still had the shore tower effort to perform when in port.

While at NOTS we fired approximately 12 missiles, and during one year aboard the USS Norton Sound perhaps 20 missiles. Not a single missile was ever lost as a result of Missile Guidance Radar malfunction. During this year, I was the Missile Guidance Radar operator.

A Field Engineer from Western Electric, producers of the Mark 25 Fire Control Radar and another from Reeves Instrument Corp. where the radar was modified, were assigned to look over our shoulder and assist us as necessary. Both these engineers were required to cover operations aboard the Norton Sound and at NOTS. They operated between both places depending upon operations. As Radar Crew Chief, I got along very well with both these individuals.

We compiled reams of data related to radar characteristics. It was soon determined we needed to improve the standing wave ratio in the wave guide run between the Transmitter/Receiver and the Antenna. This entailed removing all wave guide components and transporting them to Michaelson Lab at NOTS, China Lake. The two field engineers mentioned above went to the GMTU Officer-in-Charge, Cmdr. Slack, and told him they needed one of his men to go to NOTS with them and did not care who it was so long as it was Herriford, me. My orders were written for one week TAD, (Temporary Additional Duty). However, this stretched into three weeks before I got back to the ship. I was flown up to NOTS in a navy SNJ aircraft along with the wave guide, and wound up flying the plane for 45 minutes while the pilot dozed. Ten minutes out of Armitage Field, the Lt. took over and put us through some aerobatics. Were it not for the equipment I had on board, he would have given me a more thrilling ride.

On the return from NOTS, the operations officer on the Norton Sound, Comdr. Gay, the only surviving pilot of Torpedo Squadron 8 in the battle of Midway, needed to get his 4 hours flight time in for the month, so as to draw his flight pay, flew a Navy SNB to Armitage Field to pick me up. Riding in the copilot's seat was the ships Chief Warrant Boatswain, while the actual copilot, the Lt. who flew me up there initially in the SNJ, was back in the cabin with me. The tower gave Comdr. Gay the runway number from which to take off. However, Gay took the first runway he came to ignoring the tower. Anyway, in the take off attempt, we ran out of runway and wound up about two hundred yards out in the desert. Gay then chewed the tower out for putting him on the wrong runway. We then got onto the designated runway and became airborne. When we arrived over the Oxnard Plain, it looked like a blanket of cotton extending well out over the Pacific. Our pilot had to make an instrument approach until we descended below 200 feet. At that point, we could see the ground and hangers of Point Mugu Naval Air Station. Our pilot was slipping us right into one of the hangers until the Lt. in the cabin with me alerted the pilot of his plight. When we got on the ground, Cmdr. Gay became very irate with the Lt.

I was to have another experience with Cmdr. Gay a few weeks later. He was acting Executive Officer when I had to put one of my men on report for direct disobedience of orders. I, being a Chief Petty Officer, was called into his presence and handed a book on the management of personnel with instructions to read it and submit a book report on the subject. He rejected the report and it appeared I was the only one punished. What a character!

During the summer of 1951, Ltjg Ed Fraker reported aboard Norton Sound with orders to be placed under my tutelage for a month in order to learn the Missile Guidance Radar. He was a Chief Fire Controlman who had been advanced to his WW-II commission after the Korean conflict commenced. After leaving Norton Sound, he was to become Officer in Charge of the R and D Launch Site on G-1 Range at the Naval Ordnance Test Station, (NOTS), China Lake, California. This was the facility we of GMTU-21 had helped install and operate during our tenure there. Upon my departure from NOTS, I turned the Missile Guidance Radar over to a Civil Service Technician who apparently did not posses the ability to keep the system in operation. This individual was relieved when the station CO of Naval Personnel assigned 8 sailors under Lt Fraker to the job. Fraker knew very little about the guidance radar system and the men assigned to his supervision even less.

22

To Norfolk, Virginia

The Guided Missile Unit-21 transferred to the USS Mississippi, EAG-128, home ported in Norfolk, Virginia in early January 1952, except for me. I obtained a one month delay for several reasons, but mainly related to turning over the Missile Guidance Radar to Norton Sound technicians and making sure they could maintain and operate it. My transfer was effective on February 1, 1952, giving me about two weeks to make the trip.

Our routing took us first to Tulsa where we visited my relatives and rested up for a couple days. Then to Marion, Indiana, for two more days of rest and visits with Jaretta's parents and relatives before heading for Norfolk.

There were few places to live in Norfolk. We first took an upstairs apartment in a private home. Our landlord was a cranky old cuss who let me know from the start that he raised the best maters and taters in his garden. Shirley had a dog she had raised from a puppy. We towed a small utility trailer belonging to one the members in the Guided Missile Unit across country, with a doghouse and the dog being part of its load. The dog and doghouse were permitted to be kept in the back yard. Heat in our apartment was via registers in our floor into the room below. There was no way to regulate the heat we got, and the three rooms were very small. Privacy was almost nonexistent.

My paternal grandmother passed away 1 March, 1952, and I obtained emergency leave to return to Cleveland, Oklahoma for the funeral. Our landlord agreed to look after our dog, so Jaretta, Shirley and I headed west in the car following route US-60. All the second day we traveled in drizzling rain and it was quite cold. All across southern Missouri, I was making good time in what appeared to be a light rain doing about 60 miles an hour. About 15 miles south of Springfield, we came upon a diner and decided to have a sandwich and some coffee. Upon stepping out of the car, I nearly slipped down on my butt. There was solid sheet of ice covering everything. My heart jumped up in my throat. To think I had been driving the last two or three hours on this stuff really shook me up on top of which, it was bitterly cold.

There was nothing near the dinner. Yet I felt we should get in off the highway. Snow was beginning to come down rather heavily. A truck driver having a bite to eat told me to follow his rig when he left, that he would get us into Joplin where we should be able to get a motel. Well, we made it to Joplin, but by this time all motels and hotels were jammed full. My car heater would not put out any heat, so I obtained a road map from a shell service station, secured it across the lower portion of the radiator and we had heat. The snow had by now let up, so we headed for Tulsa, arriving there about 8:00 AM. An hour later, we were in Cleveland. Our return to Norfolk following the funeral was uneventful.

Duty aboard Mississippi proved to be quite a drudgery. This was the old battleship of World War II fame with her main battery gun turrets removed and now serving as a development platform for new weapons systems. She was designated EAG-128 operating under the command of Operational Development Force, (OPDevFor). The first Terrier Missile automatic load and launch system had been installed before my arrival on board. The usual routine was to ride a motor launch from the fleet landing at the naval base out to the ship anchored in Hampton Roads on Monday morning, arriving normally about 0700 in time for breakfast. At 0800 underway for the Virginia Capes. This required about three hours to clear out of Chesapeake Bay and get on station. While I was on board there were two projects going: One involved development and firing of **TERRIER** guided missiles and the other was firing of a 3 inch twin gun mount located just a few feet forward and one deck level below my Missile Guidance Radar room. The purpose of this firing was development of proximity fuses for antiaircraft ammunition. Those 3 inch guns are worse on the ears than any other naval gun because of their sharp crack.

Now, if the weather was good, the ship would engage in one or the other of the aforementioned exercises. However, on the other hand, if the weather was foul, the ship would anchor on a sandbar about 40 feet deep and we might just wallow there in the open sea until Friday afternoon, at which time the anchor would be recovered and we would steam back into Hampton Roads for the weekend. Believe me there is a lot of foul weather off the Virginia Capes. On one occasion, we steamed up to New York for a weekend. This was the only break in the established routine while I was aboard. At this point in time, a missile shoot could be conducted in a couple hours.

After a couple months in that small upstairs apartment, a vacancy developed at Riverdale Manor, a wartime housing facility. We jumped at the chance. It was full of cockroaches to begin with, but in no time Jaretta had eliminated them. Jaretta was an extremely clean housekeeper. We lived there about six months when a brand new apartment complex opened up. Our application was accepted and we moved again, but this time it was into a new clean two-bedroom unit. It was a pleasure to be there.

23

Back to NOTS

One morning, less than a month after our last move, I arrived on the quarter deck of Mississippi in Hampton Roads and was greeted by Lcdr Arthur Hamilton, our new Officer-in-Charge of GMU #21. He had my orders in his hand, to return to NOTS for 3 months temporary duty. He stated that my orders would most likely be extended for another 3 months of temporary duty, then it would become permanent. The Missile Guidance Radar it seemed had malfunctioned at NOTS and the assigned personnel could not get it back in operation long enough to conduct a missile shoot. I had about 45 minutes to pack all my gear and catch the last boat back to the Fleet Landing before the ship got under way.

Temporary duty orders do not allow collecting travel allowance for transfer of dependents. However, I was not about to leave Jaretta and Shirley on the east coast while I would be on the west coast for a minimum of six months. Jaretta was very surprised at my return home so early. We discussed the situation a few minutes, then called a van line to come out and pack our belongings. This was on Wednesday morning. Luck was with us. The van line had their people there right after lunch and by 5:00 PM all our things had been packed and ready for loading early next morning.

That night, I loaded most of the things we were taking in the car. The van arrived about 8:00a.m. Thursday and they were loaded and ready to roll about 9:45. We put our remaining things into the car and left sharply at 10:00 AM, California bound.

On temporary orders, I had 5 days in which to report in at NOTS commencing at 08:00 on Thursday. Thus, I had until 08:00 the following Tuesday morning to arrive at my destination. Were my orders permanent rather than temporary, I would have had 10 or 12 days to make the trip.

I drove non-stop without relief, other than stops for gas, coffee, and a sandwich arriving at my sister, Dorothy's home on Friday night about 11:00 p.m. We left there at 1:00 p.m. on Saturday and arrived at a motel in San Bernardino, California, about 2:00a.m. Monday. The portion of the trip from Albuquerque, N.M. west found me sitting on pillows resulting from a cyst on the right cheek of my butt. Upon our arrival and check in at NOTS, China Lake, I was immediately committed to the dispensary. By now I could hardly walk. Jaretta and Shirley had to find a motel for a few days on their own. Fortunately, we knew the people who owned the Inyokern Hotel in Inyokern, 9 miles west.

I was released from the dispensary after about three days and went out on G-1 Range to make my acquaintance with the problems there. After checking in with Lt. Ed Fraker, the officer in charge, I began a slow tour of the Weapons Control Center. There were 6 or 8 enlisted sailors present around the coffee mess watching me like a hawk. Without introducing myself, I continued my inspection, opening the various radar cabinets, observing the computer and looking behind the fire control switchboard.

Finally, I approached the group and inquired as to who was the senior petty officer. Having established his identity, I inquired if they ever held Field Day on any of the equipment? The reply was, "Chief, if we clean it up today the wind will blow tomorrow and it will be dirty again." At this point, I introduced myself and informed them as of that moment the order was conduct field day, and if the wind blew later, that would be followed by field day again. All electronic equipment had about a quarter inch of dust on all chassis. Further, a rat's nest was found in one of the large rotary switches when it was pulled out of the Fire Control Switchboard.

One of my first acts was to establish a two-shift operation to facilitate equipment up-keep and maintenance. A commander, don't recall his name, from the Navy Special Projects Office arrived on scene to inquire of my needs in order to get the radar back into operation. I told him I needed 30 days of uninterrupted down time. This he agreed to. My sailors turned to. First, the equipment was thoroughly cleaned up, thus making it a pleasure to work with. Second, we started through every chassis and every circuit in each of the radar cabinets to verify integrity of each circuit. In the Range Unit alone, we removed 13 illegal circuit changes installed by the civil service technician to whom I had turned the equipment over back in December 1950. Many other such changes were found throughout the remaining six cabinets of electronics.

Another problem I had to resolve: One of my petty officers informed me that when a problem occurred in the radar, Lt. Fraker had gotten into the habit of taking over the enlisted technician's job, and having the technician hand him the tools. Immediately I let Fraker understand that his position was administrative and that he was to stay away from the equipment. Solved that problem.

There was a strange organization situation within which we operated. The Terrier Guided Missile development operations on G-1 Range was under a department in Michaelson Laboratory. This department was headed up by a single individual with one civil service engineering type directly assigned to him. While we navy personnel reported to the personnel officer on the base, we reported to this department head regarding technical matters. Early on, I had to run the civil service engineer off. He had the idea he out ranked me and began to conduct tests of his own contrary to my efforts to rehabilitate the system. He was one mad engineer.

I established a maintenance program for all equipment in the Weapons Control facility and within the 30-day down period, all equipments were properly configured and operational. We were ready to shoot missiles. From that time on, we never missed a shoot nor did we ever lose a missile. Another problem was that I, being on temporary orders was not eligible for military housing on the base. This forced us to live in Inyokern. However, about November 6, a set of orders for me to go to Reeves Instrument Corp. for three months were received. This, then made my assignment to NOTS permanent, thus making me eligible for base housing, which I applied for immediately and was assigned a house. My orders required me to depart NOTS before our move to base housing could be affected. Fortunately, I had some good men in my crew and they moved Jaretta and Shirley onto the base a couple days after I left. Furthermore, they looked in on them frequently to see if they needed help of any kind. The mean part of these orders was my being in New York over the holiday season did not bode well, especially through the winter months.

24

Establish GMU-25

On Tuesday, November 11, 1952, I departed NOTS on a special flight set up for me alone, to Travis Air Force Base. At one time, the Navy had quite a number of enlisted pilots. Nearly all had held commissions during WW-II and the Korean conflict, but had reverted back to their permanent enlisted ratings. About a dozen were left in the Navy at this time, and all were assigned to NOTS. These pilots could fly anything that was designed to get into the air. Their versatility made them indispensable for the many projects being conducted at NOTS. My particular flight was in a Navy R-4D, (DC-3) manned by all enlisted personnel, the pilot being a CPO with whom I was acquainted. Flight time was about one hour and forty-five minutes to Travis AFB. After becoming airborne, the PO1/c who was copilot moved back into the cabin and I occupied his seat up front until we were about 5 minutes from touch down.

Here is an interesting true story about one of these enlisted pilots. His name was Adams, a tall skinny Chief Petty Officer who would rather fly than eat. To begin, back before Pearl Harbor when General Claire L. Chennault first formed his Flying Tigers in China, Adams an enlisted Navy pilot obtained a leave of absence from the Navy and joined the Flying Tigers. He flew with Chennault until they broke up with commencement of WW-II, at which time he was returned to Washington, D.C. By this time, he had advanced to Rank of Colonel in the Flying Tigers and the Army Air Corps. was trying to send him to

Europe as commander of a P-47 squadron. About this time, Adams threw up his hands and said, "you cannot do this to me, I'm Navy". He then got Navy Bureau of Personnel on the phone to confirm his position. Navy took him back as a LtCdr and made him a fighter squadron commander flying from aircraft carriers.

One day while I was at NCTS, Adams flew down to Ft. Bliss, Texas in an R4-D, (DC-3) to pick up a group of people who were touring various guided missile facilities, to bring them back to NOTS. While Adams and his Plane Captain were standing outside and adjacent to the boarding ladder, an Air Force Lt. Col asked Adams who was Flying this ship? Upon Adams reply that he was the pilot, the Colonel next asked who his copilot was? Adams then pointed out a Navy Lieutenant standing a few feet away. With that the Colonel then asked Adams how many hours he had in the air? Adams replied, "Oh I don't know, perhaps about 40,000 I guess". With that, the Colonel shut up and boarded the aircraft. The Plane Captain, having overheard the foregoing conversation, went to the Control Tower Chief when they returned to Armitage Field and they pulled Adams flight record. Would you believe Adams had in excess of 42,000 hours of flight time as a pilot.

The following morning, I was scheduled to fly the "Milk Run", a non-stop Military Air Transport Service, (MATS) flight to Washington, D.C. My name was the second called to board the aircraft and I felt silly as hell walking out behind a Vice Admiral. While I knew my trip and project were of high priority, it never dawned on me that it was such as to put me ahead of a congressman who followed me.

We were provided box lunches, which contained the equivalent of two lunches. The seats were all facing aft. Flight time approximated eleven hours, so with 3 time zone changes we arrived at Washington National Airport about 11:00 PM. I took a cab to the Annapolis Hotel, expecting to catch a flight on to New York the following day.

Next morning, I took a flight into La Guardia Airport, reported in at the Naval Receiving Station in Brooklyn and was sent out to the Reeves Instrument Corp. facilities at Roosevelt Field on Long Island, where I was to spend the next 3 months. To my surprise, two of my radar crewmen from GMTU-21 on the USS Mississippi had been ordered to Reeves also and were already there. The three of us rented an apartment in Long Beach. Whittington, ET1/c and Cowen FT3/c were to comprise the nucleus of my new radar gang. Again, we were each living on $5.00 a day perdiem, but by pooling these funds, we were able to pay rent and buy groceries. Cowen was the designated cook. However, we still depended on the Reeves engineers buying us lunch 5 days a week or we would have gone hungry. Whittington was with me during my first 6 months at Reeves in the winter of 1949 and 1950. However, this was Cowen's first time.

It so happened that the Civil Service Engineer whom I had previously run off the radar at NOTS managed to wrangle orders to Reeves for a couple weeks. He had previously written a letter announcing his arrival. I knew all the engineering staff at Reeves and was well received by them. When I first approached Sid Meadows, his remark to me was, "who is this SOB? Said his letter must have been composed with a Roget's Thesaurus readily at hand, and upon his arrival had tried to hand the engineering staff a snow job.

The contract to Reeves instrument Corp. was to modify a Mark 25, Mod 2 Fire Control Radar to a Mod 7 Missile Guidance Radar. Reeves engineers established classes of instruction and lectured us three Navy people on the technicalities of the new system. In turn, having considerable experience with developing and maintaining previous systems, our advice and recommendations were given utmost attention in design requirements for the new system. Again, it fell to me to write the alignment and integration procedures for the technical manuals. This was no small task. Later on it would become my responsibility to perform the integration of the entire launch system at the permanent site when I returned to NOTS.

I returned home on February 3, 1953. It was not a happy reunion. Jaretta was angry with me for having bought a couple bottles of whiskey during the winter while I was in the N.Y. area. It is true both she and Shirley also had had a rough time of it financially while I was away. It was amazing, Shirley's dog, that was just a pup when I left went wild when I returned. The dog remembered me.

We Navy people on G-1 Range had no formal organization at this time. The group developing Sidewinder, (Air-to-Air Missile) were in GMU-65. Temporarily, we in the Terrier Missile Group reported to GMU-65 situated in a large Quonset Hut behind Michelson Laboratory. There I became acquainted with the people and their efforts in development of Sidewinder. About a month later, Guided Missile Unit-25 was formed and our ranks began to increase in personnel. We topped out at about 20 sailors, including two Chief Petty Officers besides myself. Lt. Fraker had been transferred prior to my return from N.Y.

Ltjg Hensley, a reserve officer, initially became Officer-in-Charge and he was an all right individual. Had his head screwed on right. However, a short time later another Ltjg reported aboard and he was scared of his own shadow. Mr. Hensley and I practically led him by the hand most of the time. I do not remember his name, but he had time in rank on Hensley, therefore became our new Officer-in-Charge, (O-n-C). He was a likable individual despite his short comings.

GMU-25 began to grow with new personnel. It therefore became my responsibility to run Guided Missile Unit 25 in a technical sense. We were facing installation of all new equipment at a permanent launch site.

Whittington, Cowen and I moved temporarily into the Range Design section in Michelson Lab. We were set up with drafting tables and commenced preparing the system integration drawings (Blue Prints). This job was completed in about five weeks. By the time we returned to G-1 Range, foundations had been poured for the launcher and the Mark 37 Gun Director upon which the Guidance Radar Antenna would be mounted.

Several years previous when the Gun Director was installed at the temporary launch site, NOTS gave a $35,000 contract to Long Beach Naval Shipyard for two men to come to China Lake and perform the machine alignment and installation for this unit. Surprisingly, the individual who headed up this two man team was one of the civilians in my advanced Fire Control School class in Washington, D.C. Now the Department Head in Michelson Lab, for the two man department to which GMU-25 reported. asked me if I could perform this job? Said he could not provide me with any monetary compensation, but would see to it that a letter on the subject would be placed in my service record. I assured him I could accomplish the job, but that I would need the assistance of two Civil Service Outside Machinists. This he agreed to, but I am still looking for that letter.

With two of my sailors and the two Civil Service types, we commenced the effort. The Gun Director weighed in at 16 tons, and was mounted atop a barbet nine feet in diameter and eight feet high. Tolerance for concentricity of the barbette in azimuth was .003 inch on the narrow diameter and .007 inch on the wide diameter, thus allowing an ellipticity of .004 inch. This time of year, temperatures in the desert reached 115 to 120 degrees during the day. Since the sun was on one side of the barbette in the morning and the other in the afternoon, distortion of the steel in the barbette was quite pronounced. Stabilization occurred about one o'clock in the morning. That factor determined when we went to work. We had to knock off work ten minutes after the sun appeared above the horizon.

First, we had to raise the director .010 inch using timbers and jacks to let the barbette relax under the rollerpath. Eight adjustable radial thrust rollers had to be adjusted in accordance with dial indicator readings in order to establish concentricity. Then it was necessary to hand ream and mic sixteen holes for which individual body bound, hold-down bolts were machined for each hole that had to be driven home with a large hammer. The job was completed in two weeks and within all specified tolerances.

By now, GMU-25 had acquired about six new CPO's and as many new enlisted men. As senior CPO, I still had technical responsibility for the unit, including disciplinary measures from time to time. For example, one of the sailors returned from leave sporting a "duck butt haircut". I sent him to the Station Barber to have it removed. Upon his return to the Range, he still had it, whereby I ordered him into my pickup and personally took him to the barber.

We had just completed the new launch system installation when I received orders changing my rate from Chief Fire Control Technician to Chief Guided Missileman including a statement to the effect that reversion to the former rate would not be considered. This event forced me to work in the Guided Missile Assembly and Checkout Building. Although I was still senior chief, my responsibilities were turned over to another CPO. After about six weeks, I found my new job so boring that I was determined to try to get my rate reversed. Other people in the unit said I was spinning my wheels.

I sent my letter to Bureau of Personnel stating, "I could make a Guided Missileman out of any truck driver in a matter of six weeks, and that my talents in my previous rating were being wasted." I sent this letter via Capt. Bud Slack in the Bureau of Ordnance, Special Projects

Office, the former Officer-n-Charge of GMTU-21, for his endorsement. Soon as I received a copy of Capt. Slack's endorsement, everyone agreed I was a cinch to be reverted, and I was six weeks later.

My enlistment expired about this time and I shipped over for six more years. In so doing, it became necessary to transfer to another duty station or ship. There was only one place for me to go and that was to the USS Norton Sound for a second tour of duty aboard.

Jaretta and I left China Lake in April 1956, me having orders to the USS Norton Sound. Having just shipped over, I had 30 days leave plus 6 days travel, so we made a trip back to Iowa then to Oklahoma to visit, first Jaretta's parents followed by mine. I reported aboard the ship at Hunters Point Naval Shipyard. She was being outfitted with a new Mark 25, Mod 7 Missile Guidance Radar.

Although I was the senior Chief Fire Controlman in the Fox Division upon reporting aboard, various people connived to put me in charge of the ships 40mm and 5-inch gun batteries, thus keeping me away from the missile guidance radar. I went along with this arrangement for about 4 months.

The guidance radar fired only one missile shortly after coming out of the shipyard, after which it could not be brought up within the parameters necessary to launch and guide a missile to the target. From time to time when venturing into the radar spaces I noticed the Reeves and Western Electric field engineers along with the Chief Warrant Radio Electrician, the Officer-in-Charge, were always doing the work technicians should have been doing. The CPO assigned to the radar along with various of his crew had, on several occasions, complained to me about this situation. Several times I stood JOOD watches with the Chief Warrant Radio Electrician as OOD and told him that if I was assigned to that unit I would run both him and the field engineers off and would not let them come near unless I sent for them.

One Friday afternoon, I ventured into the Missile Shop and was surprised when Capt. Bud Slack shook my hand and in the process announced to all present that here was the **best radar technician in the fleet**. Slack had come out from the Bureau of Ordnance to find out why the Guidance Radar was down and no missiles were being launched. Suffice it to say the following Monday morning, I found myself assigned to the Missile Guidance Radar and a new Officer-in-Charge had been assigned.

First off, I asked the ships captain for a 30-day shutdown of the radar, which was granted. Next, both Reeves Instrument Company and Western Electric field engineers were assigned to the wardroom at my request. Then, I briefed my FCT1/c as to what I expected of him and his crew of technicians with the admonition that if they could not cut it, I could

About three weeks after I had taken over the Mark 25, Mod 7 Missile Guidance Radar, test parameters were beginning to meet requirements. The ship was making ready to get underway one morning when the Captain sent word to me that we had an important personage aboard and requested if my radar could possibly shoot a missile that day. I sent word back that I would have an answer for him within 30 minutes. My FCT/1c, Snow assured me he could get the system boresighted and felt confident we could conduct the shoot. I sent word back to Captain Chung-Hoon that we could perform a shoot as he requested. We launched a missile and never again were we unable to shoot **Terrier** missiles with my Missile Guidance Radar.

As a point of interest, Captain Chung-Hoon, up until 1956, was the only Korean to have graduated from the U.S. Naval Academy, Anapolis, MD. He was the Commanding Officer of USS Norton Sound, AVM-1 during my second tour of duty aboard that ship in 1956 and 1957.

There was however, another missile guidance radar system aboard built by Sperry Gyroscope. This system was built from the ground up as a missile guidance radar, not a modified Fire Control Radar as was the Mark 25, Mod 7, (My system). Each time this radar was scheduled to fire a missile, my system was up and ready to take over in case they could not conduct the shoot. Invariably, my system would be burdened to conduct the shoot ten to fifteen seconds before launch. I do not recall that system ever fired a missile during my tour of duty aboard Norton Sound.

The new Guidance Radar Officer, a former enlisted person, the Chief Master-at-Arms and I were standing on the boat deck one morning conversing, shortly after I had taken over the Mark 25, Mod 7 system, when the two CPO's heading up the other Guidance System Crew approached the Radar Officer requesting to speak with him. Their complaint was that I had put the word out that all personnel in the Fox Division during working hours would at all times be in working uniform unless on watch or in a duty status. This was the most top heavy division I had ever experienced, with a total of 14 CPO's, I being most senior.

These two chiefs expressed to the three of us that my orders were interfering with their primary duty of debugging and getting the other Guidance Radar up and operating. They were in the habit of letting their crew go shirtless during working hours. With this statement, both the Radar Officer and the Chief-Master-at-Arms blew their tops. First, the Radar Officer informed them in no uncertain terms that their Primary Duty was Military, and that the radar project was their Technical Duty and was Secondary. Then the Master-at-Arms climbed their frames informing them he had never had any problems with my personnel and that they had better shape up fast.

I can proudly say that with five different Missile Guidance Radar Systems at three different locations, i.e. NOTS, 2; USS Norton Sound, 2; and USS Mississippi,1; involving approximately fifty separate missile shoots, not a single missile was ever lost due to a malfunction of my equipment.

In the spring of 1957, ten terrier missiles were brought aboard which were configured for recovery following a shoot. A new radome design had been incorporated on the Terrier Guided Missile and it was necessary to find out what kind of erosion occurred during flight in inclement weather. Therefore, Norton Sound left Port Hueneme, CA for a period approximating six weeks for the Pacific side of Panama, where we fired missiles through rain squalls. An automatic rain gauge was mounted on the ship's bullnose such that we could stick the bow of the ship into a rainsquall. If the rain was coming down at a rate of 1-inch per hour or greater, we would steam 4 or 5 miles away, launch a radio controlled Target Drone, then fly it to the opposite side of the rain squall. Following this, a guided missile would be launched through the rain toward the target drone. Both missile and drone were equipped with flotation devices such that 9 missiles and 8 drones were recovered.

Norton Sound returned to Port Hueneme, CA in early September 1957, and settled into our normal routine. One afternoon, I had occasion to go into Officer Country where I encountered a Chief Warrant officer. He asked if I had seen my orders. With a negative reply from me, he then proceeded to inform me that I had been selected to Warrant Officer. I informed him that I was of a good mind to reject the advancement. However, he convinced me I should take it. Shortly thereafter, Captain Grala called me into his quarters and swore me in. He then invited Jaretta and me to a little cocktail party that evening at his quarters on the base.

Following this, I was relieved of all my duties, and moved out of the CPO Quarters into a vacant stateroom up in Officers Country. It was necessary to obtain new uniforms which took the better part of the following week during which, most of my time was spent in my stateroom completing paperwork of various requirements. Finally, my orders came in assigning me as Fire Control Gunner aboard the heavy cruiser USS Helena, CA-75.

25

Warrant Officer

Heavy cruiser USS Helena, CA-75 was in the Mare Island Naval Shipyard at Vallejo, California, undergoing her periodic three-month overhaul when I reported aboard. She had been in the yard about one month by this time, November 1957. Air hoses, power cables, and all manner of equipment littered her decks on all levels. Speaking frankly, it looked like one hell of a mess.

The first thing I did was report to the Gunnery Officer, a mustang commander of Irish decent. My first question was to whom do I report? He informed me I reported directly to him. With that I made a request which, to my surprise, impressed him most significantly. I asked would he inform all other gunnery department officers that all men in the Fox Division worked for me, and that if they had need of any of my men, they would be kind enough to clear it with me. This, the Gunnery Officer, (I cannot remember his name at the moment) readily agreed to. He was a very soft spoken individual. Ordinarily he could be heard across the table if you listened carefully. However, when he became angry he could be heard all the way to the end of the table. The Gun Boss was well liked by all who came in contact with him. He informed the department officers that the Warrant Officers in the gunnery department, namely the Boatswain, Bullet Gunner, and myself, the Fire Control Gunner all worked for him, and furthermore that any time he wanted to know what was going on he would ask his Warrant Officers.

Immediately, I established a wonderful rapport with this gentleman. Technically my title was "Warrant Ordnance Control Technician", (Later, "Chief Warrant Ordnance Control Technician"). Almost immediately upon assuming my duties, I learned that the Chief Engineer was treasurer for the overhaul funds. Shipyard personnel were doing most of the work going on in the engineering spaces while ship's company was observing. However, in the Gunnery Department 90% of the overhaul of ordnance equipment: i.e. gun and turret power drives; gun directors; computers; stable elements; and fire control radars were all being overhauled by my men in the Fox Division. I had a total of eighty-five sailors working on about 60 different tasks, altogether averaging approximately 30% completion at the time I reported aboard.

While I resented the fact that most of the overhaul funds were being spent on the engineering department, it occurred to me that a good engineering plant was necessary to get my guns where they were most effective. My people were gaining invaluable experience and knowledge of interalignment and operation of the three different gun batteries within the ship, while performing the bulk of the Fire Control Equipment overhaul...Each morning we Warrant Officers met with the Gunnery Officer to assess progress of work being accomplished in our respective areas, along with priorities for various job completion.

The 8" Main Battery and 5" Secondary Battery Plotting Rooms were 5 decks down in the very bottom of the ship directly below the forward superstructure. Their respective battery gun directors were about the highest points in both the forward and after superstructures, two directors for each battery. The ship was approximately 676 feet long with a beam of 76 feet displacing about 17,600 tons. The ship's armament comprised three 8", 55-cal triple turrets (nine guns) in the main battery; two turrets forward and one aft. Six 5", 38-cal dual purpose twin mounts in the secondary battery; and six 3", 50-cal twin mounts in the antiaircraft battery. Each of the twin 3-inch mounts had its own Mark 56 Gun Director with individual Stable Element and Fire Control Radar. My field of expertise and my responsibility was the operational readiness of these systems.

The ship was put in dry-dock for a month toward end of the yard period. For battery alignment purposes, it is necessary to measure the tilt of each roller path for each gun mount, turret, director and stable element in the ship at the time water has been admitted into the dry dock and shut off, just before the ship is buoyant enough to lift clear of the keel blocks. At this time, dry-dock flooding is ceased. At this time, Gunners Quadrants are mounted in each of the elements making up the various gun batteries. A reference plain must be selected. The forward Mark 37 secondary battery gun director became our reference plain. The Gunners Quadrants are capable of measuring angles as small as 6 seconds of arc and can be estimated to 3 seconds. Every 10 degrees of azimuth the angle of inclination is measured and plotted for each unit within the ship. From this data, the inclination and angle of bearing of the high point for each roller path can be plotted, thus permitting setting of the inclination compensator for that unit. This operation requires four to five hours to complete, plus several more hours to complete the inclination plots and set the respective inclination compensators...When finished, all elements within the ship are now set to a common horizontal reference plane. This then, is the foundation of battery alignment. Many more steps are required before the alignment is complete, i.e. electrical alignment of the remote control system, bore sighting on stars, etc.

I realize the foregoing is for most people rather boring; however, there are some who will appreciate the technicalities necessary to achieving naval gunfire accuracy. This was my responsibility.

Unfortunately, about half way through taking rollerpath data, the ship hogged, although it was not apparent to anyone until after we had completed taking our data and shipyard people again commenced flooding the dry dock. Too much water had been let into the dry dock initially and the ship came clear of the keel blocks. All our efforts and recorded data were for naught.

The result of this problem now required a Gunners Quadrant be mounted in both the Reference Director and the unit for which data need be taken after the ship is water-borne. Using battle telephone circuits, it was necessary to adjust each Quadrant by verbally calling "mark" over the phones until bubbles on both quadrants coincided. The difference of the two readings then was the inclination of that unit from the Reference Director taken every ten degrees of relative bearing in azimuth. The ship was afloat so it became extremely difficult and time consuming to obtain these data. However, we prevailed. Battery alignment was roughly complete by the time we left the shipyard two weeks later. However, it would require several more weeks of refinement such as bore sighting on stars before achieving pinpoint accuracy.

Helena was commanded by Captain James T. Lay, son-in-law of Fleet Admiral Chester Nimitz. The afternoon we left Mare Island Naval Shipyard, the Train Drive Ampladyne Motorgenerator in the forward MK 37 Gun Director failed as we were steaming down the bay, before clearing the Golden Gate. My standing orders in such an event, was to immediately affect repairs day or night, spare parts permitting. Fortunately, we did have a spare aboard and my people were in the process of exchanging the motor generator when Captain Lay appeared on the scene. The Skipper asked me point blank, why 65% of the overhaul funds were spent on the propulsion plant and only 20% on ordnance? All I could answer was that the chief engineer controlled the overhaul funds. He seemed satisfied with my answer. My sailors had the director back in operation by 2200 (10:00 PM) that evening.

26

USS Helena, CA-75

Helena's homeport was Long Beach, California. Following the yard period, it was necessary to devote six weeks with Underway Training Command operating out of San Diego to restore operational and battle efficiencies. This included all manner of emergency drills, ship handling, and gunnery exercises. While we usually returned to Long Beach on weekends, Helena often anchored Monday through Thursday night in Pyramid Cove on San Clemente Island unless night operations were scheduled. In this case, we might steam all night while undergoing various nighttime drills including shooting of a battle practice. Following Underway Training, we operated out of our home port as a component of the Third Fleet.

On the north end of San Clemente Island at Wilson Cove, the Navy was in the process of developing a vertical under water launch system for the forthcoming Polaris Fleet Ballistic Missile System. This project bore the name of "Pop-up". They were in need of waves approximating ten feet in height to wash over the launch tube at the time of missile ejection. Hence, along came heavy cruiser USS Helena, CA-75. It was necessary for the ship to steam toward the southern end of San Clemente Island, about 20-miles from Wilson Cove. Then on a course pointing toward Wilson Cove the ship would build up speed to about 32 Knots.

Captain Lay and for that matter the entire ship's company was very much concerned that this vessel of 17,600 tons could wind up on the beach. From Wilson Cove a spit of land diverges at approximately 45 degrees true for a distance of about a quarter to a half mile. This required Helena to make a turn approximating sixty degrees to starboard at high speed within a quarter mile of the beach. Should there be a failure in steering control during these runs, besides control on the bridge, both forward and after Conning Stations as well as the Steering Engine Room were manned such that any one of these stations could take control in event of a steering failure. While steering failures are not common occurrences in Naval Ships, they do occur every now and then. Helena was involved with this project for nearly two weeks wherein approximately ten such runs were made.

We were scheduled to deploy to the Far East in July 1958, to become flagship of the Seventh Fleet. About this time, the situation in Lebanon came to a crisis, and all Naval units were put on alert. We had spent the previous week tied to a pier in the Long Beach Navy Yard, taking on fuel and provisions preparatory to our departure for the Far East. At once all hands were restricted to the ship. Finally, after two days, four section liberty was granted permitting visits to the Officers, CPO, and Enlisted clubs at the Naval Station for four hours at a time. During the next four days, wives and dependants could be visited in this manner. This then was our situation when it became time for our scheduled departure for West Pac. Our sister ship USS Bremerton, CA-130, also our Cruiser Division 3 Flagship, got under way about 0900 the morning of our departure, 16 July 1958, but for some reason or another Helena was held up from getting under way until about 1400, (2:00 pm).

Both ships were scheduled to steam past San Clemente Island and fire shore bombardment exercises, and then set coarse for Hawaii. Normally, a ship has one firing practice run then must declare the next run as firing for score. Having left Long Beach ahead of us, Bremerton proceeded to fire, but after obtaining her second run score, declared that run for practice also. She then commenced a third run which, was declared as firing for score. This run was eating into time allotted to Helena. By the time we got on the range, there remained only enough time for a firing run for score. Therefore, forsaking a practice run, we declared for score and out shot Bremerton by 8 percentage points. Following these firing exercises, a course was set for Pearl Harbor, where we arrived 5 days later, having accomplished a number of emergency drills during this phase of the trip to the Far East .

27

Flagship Seventh Fleet

Upon leaving Pearl Harbor on 24 July, our base course was to Yokosuka, Japan. During this phase of our cruise, many emergency drills were conducted, including Ship Towing exercise. First Helena rigged and then towed USS Bremerton, followed by Bremerton towing USS Helena.

Yokosuka was Headquarters and home port for Seventh Fleet, where we arrived on 3 August. The seventh Fleet Flag was immediately embarked and on 18 August we set a course for Keeling, Taiwan, arriving there on 21 August and from there to Kaohsiung, Taiwan on 23 August 1958. Suffice it to say, Helena was kept on the move most of the time. During the summer of this year, the Quemoy Islands, just off the coast of China, in the Taiwan Straits, were being shelled by the Chinese Communists from the mainland with 35,000 to 42,000 rounds of artillery shells daily . These islands were occupied by Chinese Nationalists from Taiwan. It so happened there was one approximately 8 inch gun on the mainland in a concrete bunker that counter fire from the islands could not take out.

The Seventh Fleet Flag provided their only chart of the Quemoy area to my Gunnery Officer, LtCdr Denny, with instructions to him and me to come up with a plan for our 8-Inch Main Battery guns to take this gun emplacement out while Helena remained on the 10 fathom curve according to the chart provided. The referent chart was dog-eared and bore much evidence of having been well handled over a good number of years. Yet, it was the only chart Seventh Fleet had of the area. After much studying of the chart, the big gun location with respect to the 10-fathom curve, proved to be about maximum effective range for our 8-Inch guns.

We then found a target rock in a chain of small islands in the Yellow Sea. Helena stood off at 26,000 yards with one of our helicopters over the island spotting for us. Not a single hit was scored on the rock during several 9-gun salvos. It was with considerable disappointment that we returned to Keelung.

Helena departed Keelung on Sunday morning 31 August 1958, about 0100, having embarked about 50 correspondents from various publications around the world. We joined a convoy of Chinese Nationalists ships re-supplying Quemoy. From dawn until dusk that day, we sat on the 10 fathom curve off the China Mainland waiting for that big gun to open up. Our objective was to take it out with our 8 inch main battery. They apparently realized why we were there and did not fire a single round that day. The ship was at General Quarters throughout the long, long day, just waiting.

This day proved to be a red-letter day for air-to-air guided missiles. The Chinese Communists had 36 aircraft in the air covering our operation. The Chinese Nationalists under Chang Kai-shek on Taiwan was equipped with F-86 fighters armed with Sidewinder heat-seeking guided missiles, with which I was well acquainted. The Chinese Nationalists sent up 18 F-86's against 36 Mig-15's. Two Sidewinder's were fired which went right up the tail pipe of their respective targets. After this, the Chi-Com's pan-caked the remaining 34 Mig's, thus ending that threat for the balance of the day. This was the first time Sidewinder Guided Missiles were fired in anger.

We rendezvoused with fleet tanker USS Cimarron south of Taiwan to refuel. As we approached on her port quarter, Cimarron lost steering control and commenced veering to starboard. Captain Lay executed a beautiful job of following, avoiding colliding until Cimarron regained control and attempted to return to base course instead of settling on the course to which she had swung. Helena's bow by this time was just abaft the island superstructure of Cimarron and she was by now cutting across our bow. Somehow, Captain Lay gave commands that caused Helena's bow to veer away with only a slight impact, but Cimarron's attempt to again steer to starboard caused her stern to swing into Helena's Starboard side adjacent to main battery turret number two. I was up in the Forward Fire Control Station above the bridge watching all this action.

While it was evident a collision was going to occur, the lapsed time of two or three minutes observing the ships come together and knowing at the same time nothing could prevent it happening, was awesome. Plates on Helena were broken and buckled for over 100 feet on three deck levels from Turret 2 forward. It did not, however, keep us from our operating schedule. Approximately ten days later when we did return to Yokosuka, all the pre cut and formed new plating, was lying on the pier when we tied up. Japanese workmen were rigging scaffolds and making efforts to remove damaged plates even before the special sea detail was secured.

Within 36 hours, all the damaged plates had been removed from three different deck levels. At this time, Seventh Fleet received news that the Chi Coms were again shelling Quemoy Islands. Many valves had been removed in the engineering spaces and were in the shipyard for repair and overhaul. Commander Seventh Fleet asked the shipyard Superintendent how long it would take to get Helena ready for sea. He gave an answer of 72 hours, whereupon Seventh Fleet gave him 36 hours. Temporary plating was secured over our starboard side. Operating on two of four engines with half our boilers inoperative, we steamed to sea within 36 hours. Twelve knots was our maximum speed. We went to Keelung, Taiwan and operated in the area for three weeks before returning to Yokosuka to finish our repairs.

Both Helena and Bremerton were in Subic Bay, Luzon, Philippine Islands, when we received word that Chinese merchant ship Hoy Wong had run upon Bombay Reef, about the middle of the South China Sea. Helena, in addition to our own, took aboard Bremerton's helicopter and we proceeded to accomplish the largest such rescue operation of its kind until that time. Hoy Wong had about 130 people on board when she ran almost full length, perhaps 350 feet upon the reef. Our small boats could get close to her stern and managed to remove only about 10 people, but it was considered too hazardous to continue this operation. The helicopters could carry only six passengers at a time and they could not land on deck of the Hoy Wong. Therefore, using a basket on a winch line, each chopper made approximately10 round trips, thus removing about 120 people that we then took to Hong Kong.

Toward the latter part of our deployment, we visited seven different Japanese cities where the Commander Seventh Fleet called upon various prefecture governors, termed good will visits. At Osaka, it was my privilege to visit Takaraska, the famous all girl academy of dance and acting. There are three different troupes approximating 100 girls each, one in residence, one in Tokyo, and one on world tour. These girls spend their entire lives with this organization, becoming instructors when they become too old to dance and act. Takaraska provided the troupe, which appeared in the movie "Sayonara" with Marlon Brando. It was a most enjoyable experience, although it was cold and there were patches of snow on the ground. Public buildings do not have central heating in the Orient. While it was very cold, the experience was most enjoyable.

We also made formal official visits to Hong Kong and to Manila. In Hong Kong, there was a tea party on the forecastle in honor of the Governor General and several of his guests. It was mandatory for all ship's officers to attend. This then, was followed by a reception given by the Governor General, which again, all Helena Officers were required to attend.

Navy regulations at that time did not require Warrant Officers to possess a sword. It was my luck however, to be Officer of The Deck, (OOD) in Kobe, Japan, when we were expecting a formal visit of the local Prefecture Governor. The Executive Officer ventured upon the Quarter Deck and asked, "Mr. Herriford, where is your sword?" I told him I did not possess one. He had a junior officer nearby relieve me long enough to go below and borrow one. When I returned he gave me two weeks to purchase my own. This I did and wore it only once thereafter.

Helena was relieved as Flagship Seventh Fleet by heavy cruiser USS Saint Paul, CA-73. On 4 February 1959, Helena set a course for Long Beach, California. We lost a day upon crossing 180 degrees of longitude. At ship's speed approximating fifteen knots, eleven days after leaving Yokuska Naval Shipyard, Japan, with no sight of land in between, we moored the ship to pier E adjacent to Long Beach Naval Ship Yard, California, about 1800 on 16 February. Distance traveled approximated 4,095 nautical miles or 4,840 statute miles.

About this time, Helena was awarded the battle efficiency pennant for her class of ship, the first time she had held this distinction since 1947, and she won it again the following year also. This permitted painting of a big white "E" on the forward stack for all to see. I feel my efforts, i.e. Battery alignment, maintenance efforts, and personnel training was largely responsible for receiving the Battle Efficiency Pennant.

Furthermore, I have certificates commemorating this fact for the years 1958 and 1959.

We were assigned to the First Fleet and operated up and down the West Coast. "Operation Pop-up" was being developed at Wilson Cove on San Clemente Island for the purpose of developing a launch system for the Polaris Missile from submerged submarines. They needed generation of a big wave to wash over the launcher at time of ejection. Helena was selected to generate the required wave. From a position near the south-east point of San Clemente Island about twenty miles from Wilson Cove, Helena would steam at flank speed, 32 Knots toward the launch facility. It was necessary for the ship to make a 65 degree turn about a half mile off shore in order to miss the point of land North-East of Wilson Cove. This was touchy business with 17,600 tons of pig iron bearing down on a land mass at 32 knots, approximately 36 1/2 miles per hour. Every available rudder control station in the ship was manned in the event a failure might occur at primary control. Imagine the concern of the Commanding Officer. For that matter, all aboard were concerned about the possibility of piling the ship on the rocks. Ten to twelve foot waves washed over the Pop-up Launcher, generated by our action. This went on for two weeks.

About this time, I started thinking about my next duty station, what I would like to be involved in, where I would like to go, etc. I had been following events related to the Polaris missile program. Having spent 9 1/2 years in the Bumble Bee program developing the Terrier Guided Missile and related Missile Guidance Radar, it struck me that I would like to get involved with Polaris. With my past experience in the missile field, I should fit right in. Having this thought in mind, I called the Warrant Officer assignment desk in BuPers and was told there was nothing available at the moment. However, the following day, I received a call from them telling me of a billet in the Polaris Program and they thought I would be the right person for it. All this transpired the early part of June 1959.

28

Polaris Program

The ship made a trip to Portland, Oregon, to participate in the Rose Festival. I received orders when we returned to Long Beach. Everyone was dumbfounded by them, including myself. Upon being detached from USS Helena the last part of June, I proceeded to carry out my orders. First, I was required to report to Inspector of Ordnance, Lockheed Missile and Space Company, Sunnyvale, California. Lockheed was Prime Contractor for Polaris. My orders required I spend 2-weeks there for indoctrination. Jaretta and I resided in a motel room during this period. My orders authorized travel by personal automobile. One day while at Lockheed, I was directed to fly in a Lockheed airplane to Sacramento, CA for a visit to the Aerojet General Plant near there. Aerojet General was the source for solid fuel rocket motors for Polaris.

My second intermediate duty station was the General Electric Ordnance Plant in Pittsfield Massachusetts for a 2-week stay. G.E. was contractor for the guidance system used in Polaris. I received a two-week crash course in ballistic missile guidance. This was a very intense subject.

We (Jaretta and I) arrived in Pittsfield during the height of the Tanglewood Music Festival. There were eight or ten different venues in the western part of the state, with people from all over the world. The result of all this was no hotel or motel accommodations were available and tickets to all venues were unavailable; they were sold out. After much searching we finally found accommodations in a large tourist lodge including meals, in Lee, MA, about 10 miles south of Pittsfield.

My orders next took me to Washington, D.C. where I reported to the Special Projects Office in the U,S, Navy Bureau of Ordnance. There I spent a week being apprised of various classified and technical requirements for operation of the Polaris assembly and checkout facility under construction at the Naval Ammunition Depot, Charleston, S.C. Everything related to Polaris was classified Top Secret.

After leaving Washington, we drove to Camp LeJeune, N.C. where our Daughter, Shirley and Son-n-law Don Ryba lived. Don, a Master Sergeant was stationed at the Marine Corps Base. Jaretta was going to stay with them while I completed my fourth and final intermediate duty station at Cape Canaveral, Florida, for a period of three weeks, before reporting to my permanent duty station in Charleston S.C.

Upon our arrival in Camp LeJeune, we had quite a shock when our daughter, Shirley informed us our eldest granddaughter, Jodee Lee had become a victim of Polio. Jodee, only eleven months old was paralyzed from the hips down. At this time, (July 2003) Jodee is 45 years old, walks on crutches with braces on both legs or is in a wheel chair. Do not ever imply that she is a cripple, she will tell you in short order that she is handicapped, but not cripple. It is something to see her get around. She does everything anyone else does. Perhaps not the same way, but gets the job done.

A day or two later, I boarded a train bound for Cape Canaveral, Florida. There I met up with Captain Harry Cox, a nuclear physics engineer in the Navy Engineering Corps, who was to be my Commanding Officer at Naval Weapons Annex, (NWA/Polarisville), Naval Ammunition Depot, Charleston, S.C. The two of us spent the next three weeks observing Polaris missile assembly and checkout, along with introduction to various missile launch facilities.

The USS Observation Island, a Navy Geophysics Research vessel, was commanded by Captain Bud Slack, formerly my boss, as Officer-in-Charge of Guided Missile Training Unit 21. A shipboard launch tube was installed on the Observation Island. Captain Slack invited Captain Cox and me to come aboard to witness the first shipboard launch of a Polaris Missile. We each were presented with Parchment Certificates commemorating this event. Subsequently, Captain Slack became the first Commanding Officer of the USS Boston, a heavy cruiser, after she had been converted to the Navy's first Guided Missile Cruiser, CAG-1. Captain Cox and I were both quartered at Patrick Air force base during our three week stay at Cape Canaveral. Following this, we each proceeded to our ultimate duty station at Charleston, S.C. Actually, I returned to my Daughter and Son-n-laws Quarters at Camp LeJeune, N.C. From there, Jaretta and I drove to Charleston, arriving there on 3 September, 1959. We rented a nice little house in North Charleston, about a mile from the Naval Shipyard, but it was a 17 mile drive to the Ammunition Depot.

The Naval Weapons Annex was under construction, about 30 percent complete when we arrived. Roadways were built up, but not yet blacktopped. Captain Cox and I were the first Staff Officers to arrive for the Naval Weapons Annex. Therefore, I headed up the Weapons Department for the following two months until the Commander, head of this department, arrived on Station. Captain Cox made me his liaison for the construction site. This required me to make a trip to that area two or three times a week, reporting status and progress to the captain. One afternoon I received a telephone call to go to the construction site and investigate a dozer driver having been run over by his own tractor.

The Rocket Motor Checkout building was being built in a swamp where water was 4 to 6 inches deep. First, all sugar pine trees had to be cleared out, using D9 Caterpillar bull-dozers. These tractors were doz-ing down sugar pines 50 to 65 feet tall and pushing them into a large pile to be burned. One of these trees flipped back over from the pile and was falling back on the dozer as it was slowly backing away. Seeing this, the driver jumped off his D-9 Cat. With the dozer slowly backing toward the Cooper River, the driver then worked his way through the muck to the rear of the tractor and stepped upon the drawbar. In reach-ing up to the back of the seat, his hand and foot both slipped off and down he went under the Caterpillar. Lucky for the driver, the dozer blade was raised about 18 inches and passed over him without injury. Because of the swamp, muck was about 2-feet deep where these tractors had been operating. The operator was rescued from the muck by his brother who was his construction boss.

Lockheed engineered the design for the Missile Assembly Building which was nearing completion at the time Navy Personnel moved in, in what was known as "Joint Occupancy" with construction people. . In early March 1960, there was no heat in the building. I found myself wearing an overcoat and overshoes throughout the day to stay reason-ably warm.

With exception of myself, all navy personnel in the Missile Assembly Building were qualified Nuclear Powered Submariners. These people, approximately 30 under my supervision, were responsible for assembly and performed the final tests of A1P Polaris Missiles prior to their being delivered dockside for installation in the submarines. Sixteen missiles comprised a ship-fill. However, it was necessary to have a backup ship-fill ready, (32 missiles) each time a vessel came in for out-loading.

Polaris had a Triple A Priority, the highest. We were working 16 hours daily, 7 days a week in order to meet schedule, although we did not start until 12:00 noon on Sunday. One night about 8:00 p.m., we ran out of a special flame retardant compound. The only source for this material was a firm in Los Angeles, California. It had a shelf life of 54 days. It was necessary for me to place a telephone call to a representative in Jacksonville, Florida, who called his firm in Los Angeles to verify they had one gallon on the shelf. I then informed him to place a hold on it and that I would inform him later with delivery instructions. Next, I called the Special Projects Office in Washington, D.C. They, in turn, arranged an 8F2U Navy fighter aircraft to fly from Mira Mar Naval Air Station near San Diego, CA to Las Alamitos Naval Air Station near Long Beach, CA where the potting compound was loaded aboard. The flight then continued to Charleston S.C. with a stop in Memphis, Tennessee for fuel. This material was in my hands by 8:00a.m. the following morning, (12 hours lapsed time).

Admiral Arleigh (31 Knot) Burke was Chief of Naval Operations during 1955 to 1961. He, along with Rear Admiral William F. "Red" Rayborn, believed the Navy should have an intermediate range ballistic missile that could be launched from the sea. Rayborn became "Father Of Polaris". At his first meetings with various PHD's and company CEO's, when he proposed mating a ballistic missile with a submarine, one PHD expressed his view that this combination was entirely incompatible. Admiral Rayborn then replied "Doctor, in the Navy we have an elixir that makes it compatible; *it is known as sweat".*

When Admiral Burke appointed Rayborn to head up the Polaris program, he issued a memorandum known as "Red Rayborn's Hunting License", permitting Rayborn to "kidnap" personnel from any other Navy job. Rayborn was further authorized to get any 45 officers in the Navy he desired for his project.

Admiral Rayborn came into the Missile Assembly Building one day and engaged me in conversation about my operation. We talked for 15 or 20 minutes when he finally stated,: "Art, we are going to put Polaris on station, on schedule, if we have to walk over the bodies of 5 of your men in doing so". We kept that commitment in September of 1960, when the first Polaris Missile submarine, USS George Washington, having been loaded with 16 ballistic missiles, proceeded on the first 90-day submerged patrol. The USS Patrick Henry followed, while the third submarine was the USS Abraham Lincoln.

29

The Naval Weapons Annex

The missile test equipment used at the Naval Weapons Annex, (NWA) was manufactured by Northrop Corporation in Anaheim, California. The equipment known as DATICO was controlled by a punched tape, programmed to perform about 200 tests on an assembled Polaris missile, was capable of printing out the results of each test. All tests were sequential and automatic unless a failure occurred, at which time testing would stop. There was a DATICO on each of the three assembly lines in the Missile Assembly Building. Such equipment required Northrop Corp, (now Northrop-Grumman Corp.) to provide engineers for support, of which there were normally three besides their resident engineer, and very often two or three visiting engineers.

Usually, I was present during missile assembly and test operations. Therefore, I became acquainted with most of these people. Many Lockheed engineers were always around, and I had worked with them all at one time or another. In the course of activating the NWA, it had fallen my lot to accomplish several very difficult and hazardous jobs that were observed by these same people. Consequently, my talents were relayed to their managers. Any number of times I was told that when I retired from the Navy, they had a job for me.

Lockheed, being the prime contractor for Polaris, designed the entire Naval Weapons Annex, (NWA). They, therefore, thought in the beginning they were going to operate the facility. Instead, the Navy informed them Navy Personnel would be operators, but that Lockheed would provide engineering staff to look over the shoulders of navy personnel. About 130 engineering types, including support staff under the management of a Mr. John Quinn, comprised the Lockheed contingent.

Subcontractors were General Electric for the missile guidance system who had 15 or 20 engineers. Aerojet General for solid rocket motors had 10 or 12 engineers. Northrop who had the missile test/checkout equipment had about 7 engineers present.

Mr. John Quinn, Manager of Lockheed Operations, often took my word on various technical requirements over that of his engineers, and when I retired from the Navy he remarked to me that if I ever needed a job to come see him. Lockheed offered me a job just prior to my retirement that was comparable to the offer made by Northrop Corporation. I accepted Northrop's offer because it was located on the West Coast, whereas Lockheed's position would have been at New London, CT and I wanted nothing to do with anything east of the Mississippi River. I was a Test Equipment Engineer with Northrop and Lockheed would have picked me up as a Field Engineer

On one occasion during a luncheon, when we got together with civilian management and Naval officers, Captain Cox delighted in getting Mr. John Quinn and myself together, then ask me to state my rate of production. When I stated I was producing a missile per-assembly line per-day, Mr. Quinn stated "Art, you cannot make that kind of production because the facility was designed for a rate of a half missile per-line per-day. What Mr. Quinn did not consider was that I was working Naval personnel, not unionized civilians. My people were capable of doing any job there was on the missile. When they completed one job, they immediately picked up on the next requirement. There was no necessity in waiting for a civilian union type in some trade to be scheduled for particular a job. By the time I retired from the Navy, we had assembled and checked out approximately 85 Polaris A1P Missiles.

Captain Cox set up a review of Missile Assembly personnel for my retirement ceremony. That was one of the most difficult occasions of my naval carrier. I was near tears during this entire review. After all, I was leaving behind approximately 21 years of naval service, the likes of which was unique in many instances.

Always there was some challenge such that no two days were alike. I loved every bit of this. While there were good days and bad days, I would not trade a single one of them for any other. Not one person in a thousand in the naval service, or for that matter even in civilian life, has ever been exposed to the broad spectrum of experience that my Naval Career presented.

My understanding of a person going into retirement should first off purchase a new car. This I did by buying a new 1960 Oldsmobile and it proved to be a smart thing to do. Jaretta and I left North Charleston, S.C. the morning of December 1, 1960, with our new car very heavily loaded. First, we went down to the U.S. Marine Corps Base at Parris Island, S.C. where our Daughter and family lived, our Son-in-Law being a drill instructor at the marine boot camp. We spent a couple days enjoying them and the grandchildren prior to heading west to California.

My new job with Northrop was slated to commence on December 14, 1960. Our household possessions had been packed up and shipped the day before we left North Charleston. After leaving our kids at Paris Island, Jaretta and I proceeded to Davis City, Iowa, for a short visit with her parents. Her father was terminal with cancer and there was no telling how much longer he had to live. I know she would have loved to have stayed for his remaining days, but my new job beckoned and it was necessary to establish an income. That visit was the last time Jaretta saw her father alive. He passed away on January 19, 1961, and while she returned for his funeral, it was not possible for me to go having just started a new job.

From Davis City we journeyed south to Tulsa. After spending two days with my mother, sisters and brother, it was necessary for us to head for California. Both Jaretta and I had hopes of acquiring a house and moving in before my having to start work. Being wintertime however, the weather caused us to have to detour south from Santa Rosa to Las Cruces, New Mexico, thus we arrived in Anaheim late the day before I was to commence work. As it turned, out I contacted Dick West, my supervisor to be and arraigned that I would not start until the following Monday, this being Wednesday. We found out that our household effects had arrived and we sorely needed a place to move them into. Would you believe we found a real estate agent who sold us a house in Garden Grove and we moved in on Saturday, December 17, 1960.

Nortronics had a contract to design and build automatic test equipment for checkout of the Polaris Fleet Ballistic Missile in the submarines in which they were loaded for patrol. To commence with, having been hired as a Test Equipment Engineer, my work consisted of assembly, debugging and functional testing of this missile checkout equipment to be installed in the submarines. I also designed automatic Go, No-Go test equipment for subassembly testing of various electronic components in the manufacturing facility.

In February 1961, I was sent down to the NWA at Charleston, S.C. where I had retired from the Navy the previous November 30, 1960. The purpose of which, was to install a modification kit in the DATICO units used to checkout the Polaris Missiles once they were assembled. I was not too well received at the NWA upon my return. After all, now I was just another civilian.

The early part of March 1961, I was sent to Cape Canaveral, Florida for 30 days in order to permit a couple engineers at the Polaris Flight

Test Facility to take vacations and also to install some modifications in the DATICO. Another Northrop engineer came on board also. The two of us were required to implement the aforementioned modifications as well as support flight test operations conducted by Lockheed, by operating the DATICO.

We got into deep trouble with the Lockheed Test Conductor on one occasion, when after working all night modifying the DATICO, we went out for breakfast. As it turned out, a flight test rehearsal had been scheduled for this particular morning, but word of this had not been relayed to us. The Test Conductor commenced ranting and raving and chewing us out. I then surprised everyone present including myself by snapping back, telling him to calm down and discuss the matter in a civilized manner. Surprisingly, he did, even though his attitude was supported by a very bloated ego. Most people disliked working with him. The Northrop personnel present, later indicated they were happy that I had the guts to stand up to this guy.

Sometime after my return to the Northrop plant in Anaheim, California, I was sent to the Lockheed facility in Mountain View, California, for a period of 8 weeks where environmental tests were conducted on a designated system to be installed in submarines. Every two weeks, we were permitted to fly home for the weekend. Following this period, our contract was beginning to taper off for engineering types. Manufacturing took over for production of the test systems we had designed and many of our engineers terminated and went to North American Aviation who had just recently landed the Apollo Program as Prime Contractor. I was asked to make that same move, However I stayed with Northrop another 6-months, until they laid me off. I had spent about 4 ½ years with Northrop Corporation, now Northrop Gruman. As it turned out, I left Northrop on a Friday and went to work for North American the following Monday morning.

30

Phoenix Program

Upon my departure from North American Rockwell, Autonetics Division, one engineer told me to stay away from Hughes Aircraft unless I had a degree. However, that was one of the first places I went. I interviewed with a couple supervisors who offered a job and I waited and waited. These people called every week wanting to know when I was going to report for work. Finally, after two months Hughes Personnel sent a letter stating openings were being held only for those of their employees facing lay off.

The next six months found me kicking over every stone in Orange County to no avail. The Aerospace business and Industry in general was beginning a slump in 1969 that lasted into 1972. There was no work to be had anywhere. Finally, after six and a half months, I decided to look in the far reaches of Los Angeles County. The very first day I applied at Hughes Aircraft Company in El Segundo, and upon my return home that day, it was on a Thursday, I received a phone call from Hughes Aircraft wanting to know if I would mind working in Culver City. To say the least, I was very elated. The drive to El Segundo was 41 Miles from my home, and considering I had been out of work for 6 1/2 months, an extra 6 miles to Culver City was music to my ears. My résumé had been sent to Mr. Earl Pay who was looking for someone having a Guided or Ballistic Missile background. Fortunately, I possessed both. I was told a Mr. Paye would most likely call me early the following week to set up an interview. To my surprise, he called me that same afternoon and set up an interview for the next day, Friday at 11:00 am. My audience with Mr. Paye and several of his subordinates took the full hour and when I left Mr. Paye asked if I could start a week from the following Monday.

Most of my first week at Hughes was devoted to indoctrination, obtaining secret clearance and becoming acquainted with people I would be working with, along with the job I was expected to perform. I was assigned to the Computer Development Laboratory, Data Systems Division, of Aerospace Systems Group, located at that time in Building 12, Culver City, California. Aerospace Systems Group comprised two divisions namely Data Systems Division and Radar Systems Division. The latter had the contract for the radar system to be installed in the Navy's new Standoff Strike Fighter aircraft F-14 being built by McDonald-Douglas.

Radar Systems contracted for the Computer Lab of Date Systems Division to design and fabricate a ground support set of test equipment having the title of Computer Test Station. The objective of this 4-bay station was to slave the same tactical computer that flew in the F-14 Aircraft, and possess the capability to independently test and fault isolate each of 4 major boxes comprising the Computer Subsystem along with two other boxes comprising the Missile Interface Subsystem of the F-14 Weapons Control System. Between two and three thousand tests were performed on each of these units.

My job therefore, was to design computer compatible circuitry capable of performing stand-alone testing of these two units comprising the aircraft to missile interface. Six guided missile stations, exclusive of two Sidewinder stations on each wing tip, were capable of accepting three different types of guided missiles, (later increased to 4 types) with each type having a peculiar I.D. signal that must be recognized by the onboard Weapons Control System in the aircraft. Suffice it to say the

F-14 could carry a mix of four different types of guided missiles, launch them all at six separate targets within a matter of less than one minute and then leave the area.

In order to test these various Large Replaceable Units, (LRU"s) it was necessary to simulate as many as 200 input stimuli simultaneously while monitoring in some cases, as many output signals. Testing involved both pass as well as failed modes of operation. All but one of these LRU's could each be tested through approximately 2500 test routines in a matter 10 or 12 minutes since all their circuitry was purely digital logic. The remaining unit however, took the better part of an hour to an hour and ten minutes to perform approximately the same number of tests. This was my number one responsibility since it was the "Logic and Timing Unit", interfacing with the six different missile stations. This unit provided necessary time delays of both short and long duration for powering up each missile while supplying various input stimuli in a precise timed sequence. Many of the simulated signal inputs consisted of variable frequencies and amplitudes, all of which were automatically applied and monitored at very precise times by the computer program I specified. All missiles on the aircraft could be powered up in about two minutes in flight. Testing the 720 Unit was a different matter however, in that it was necessary to certify all tests in both pass and fail modes for each missile station separately. Furthermore, this unit provided the launch sequence timing which varied for each of the four missile types in time duration, number of different input signals, and the timed sequence of application. The longest sequence was less than 1.3 seconds, during which time all target information to the missile was upgraded, verified and all critical functions were given a final test prior to launch.

I realize that much of the foregoing will mean little or nothing to non-technical readers. There are going to be some readers though having technical backgrounds that will appreciate the detail. My engineering experience was in large degree considered to be pioneering in the field of Guided Missiles, Ballistic Missiles, as well as both electro-mechanical analog and digital Computers…I was functioning there in the infancy of these developments.

Seven other engineers and I were assigned various sections of the Computer Test Station. We were known as the Functional Design Engineers for the station. The prototype model was designed and fabricated in one year. While we realized many improvements were necessary this system was demonstrated to the Navy and passed with flying colors.

The F-14 computer was the heart of the system. It possessed eight thousand, (8K) of twenty-four bit words of random access memory, (RAM). An external unit contained another 24-thousand words of non-destructible, sputtered-glass memory in which the Tactical Program for the F-14 was situated. That program had to be loaded into this unit by the Computer Test Station from a magnetic tape and then tested by the Computer Test Station for correctness of content. A comparison of this system to today's state of the art is almost unbelievable. For instance, I provided very precise English language inputs to my Programmer. He, in turn, converted my requirements to Octal Format, which then required manually punching these data into the computer memory via a numerical keyboard. Then followed hours and sometime days of debugging the program until it was right.

Most of the circuitry I designed was contained in a vertical drawer containing 4 each 150 dip and 4-each 180 dip Augat wire-wrap component boards. A dip constituted a location that permitted plugging in 16-pin and 14-pin micro logic chips. Off board communication was provided via 16-pin wire connectors and the drawer wiring harness.

The wire list for this drawer alone was a stack of 8 1/2 by 11-inch sheets stacked 13 inches high representing approximately 10,000 wires.

When Radar Systems contracted the Computer Lab to design the Computer Test Station, they also provided funding initially for lab engineers to support the station for two years because of the sophistication of the system. The sophistication and state of the art for this station was stated to be the equivalent of the Weapon Control System in the F-14 aircraft. As it turned out, Radar Systems continued to fund support of Lab engineers for a total of 12 years and I was the last one of the original design engineers in this capacity. A total of thirty-four systems were fabricated and delivered to the Navy.

Charlie Fears, brother of Tom Fears, both of whom played professional football with the Rams, was my Chief Project Engineer. On one occasion, Charlie presented me with the task of generating and writing design requirements for a peculiar test fixture for testing the internal power supply for a new version of the F-14 Computer. Control Data Corporation in Minneapolis designed the computer. It was, therefore, their responsibility to design and fabricate the test fixture to my design requirements.

As luck would have it, it became my responsibility to coordinate this effort with Control Data Corp. I had to make two trips back to Minneapolis in mid-winter, once in early December and the other in early February. Temperature there the first trip was 3 degrees below zero whereas the second trip it was down to19 degrees below zero.

Bob Rogers and I were the two remaining original Functional Design Engineers left on the station after 4 years. Our department manager referred to us as the Gold Dust Twins. We had an inside track on obtaining Advanced Engineering Change Notices and had developed a rapport with a couple engineers in Radar Systems who would push changes we desired through the change board. The result of this was that we effectively had our engineering change requirements firmed up and on paper by the time approval was received. All that remained was to submit our paperwork.

Flight testing and evaluation of the Phoenix Missile System for the F-14 was being conducted at Point Mugu Naval Air Station, about 65 miles up the coast from the Los Angeles area. One of our Computer Test Stations was stationed there to support these operations. It required that Bob Rogers or I or sometimes both were required, from time to time, to make a trip up there. On one such occasion, we flew up in a company aircraft. The day before Bob called his programmer, who did not like to fly and told him to volunteer for the trip or he, Bob, would call his programmer's boss and he would have to go regardless. The next morning we reported to the flight line and boarded a 4 place Beach Bonanza. Bob's programmer was quite nervous and all was well until shortly after takeoff, the pilot reached to trim the throttle with a hand that was shaking so badly he could hardly grasp it. I thought the programmer would come unglued. The pilot was afflicted with some sort of palsy, but it did not detract from his ability to fly an airplane. Point Mugu Naval Air Station was conducting flight operations that required us to circle out over the ocean for 20 minutes before getting clearance to land. Bob's programmer was most unhappy. He was faced with the return flight back to Culver City later that afternoon.

At this point, I would like to digress for a little review of electronics, which was my privilege to work with during my career. When I first entered the Navy the only vacuum tube controlled system was the power drives for the Mark 6 Stable Element and Searchlights in the latest Destroyers.

Then came Fire Control Radar followed by the Amplidyne power drive for 40mm gun mounts. These items used many vacuum tubes per system, sometimes referred to as "Bottles". Such systems were utilized throughout WW-II and well into the 1980's. Guided Missiles came upon the scene toward the end of the 1940's decade. Rule of thumb dictated an increase of one nautical mile in range for every pound of reduction in missile weight. Therefore, the advent of sub-miniature vacuum tubes. These items were about the diameter of a lead pencil and approximately one-inch long.

The latter 1950's decade saw the development of Transistors. To facilitate control circuitry, often times an entire printed circuit board approximating 2 1/2 by 4 inches was required on which to construct various control circuits containing 10 to 12 transistors plus necessary diodes, resisters, and capacitors. In the mid 1960's, these same circuits were reduced to micro chips and packaged in hermetically sealed 14 and 16 pin packages approximately 3/8 by 1 inch in size. Next came large-scale integration where entire registers or counters or timers and the like were incorporated on a single chip. These were followed by very large scale integration which incorporate entire systems such as micro-processors. Today, there are immense systems on a single chip, i.e. the Pentium-II chip which is the heart of desktop or personal computers.

When the Computer Test Station was initially designed, there was no such thing as a standard interface for various electronic instrumenta-tion, such as remotely controlled digital multimeter, precision timer, oscilloscope, printer, tape deck, etc. Therefore, the station was designed, hard wired if you will, to the peculiar interface of various state of the art instrumentation available at that time. Several years later, this posed a problem. When it became time to up-grade the system, all new test instrumentation was manufactured with a standard interface that permitted connection to a common buss for control. Each new instru-ment had a peculiar digital address code that permitted the computer to provide it with instructions over the common control buss without interfering with other instruments connected to this same buss. This became the problem however, for the younger generation of Computer Test Station engineers who came upon the scene after we older types had moved on.

When it came time to upgrade the Computer Test Station with state-of-the-art instrumentation, installation of the Instrumentation Control Buss, many cables and rack harnesses had to be physically rewired. All these changes had to be affected however, without disrupting any of the approximately 14,000 computer controlled test routines. Suffice it to say, I was consulted many times on this subject during approximately eighteen months of this project.

Reorganization of the Aerospace Division resulted in moving from Culver City. Radar systems went to El Segundo on Imperial Highway and Electro-Optical and Data Systems Group, (EDSG) containing the Computer Development Lab, moved to the most southeastern corner of El Segundo where we had a brand new manufacturing facility. I was asked to transfer to the Radar Systems Group but declined to leave the Computer Lab. Subsequently, EDSG's main mission was shifted to Space Sensors, spy-in-the-sky stuff and the Computer Lab was taken over for deep space projects. I lost all perspective of what was going on because of the need to know aspect.

Although I was from time to time called to Radar Systems in support of the Computer Test Station, and in fact, spent about three months there on temporary assignment on one occasion, I was still being assigned deep space job assignments. One such task was to design load bank requirements for a set of circuitry presented to me. Naturally, I assumed load testing for worst-case conditions. I completed the job in about six weeks and was informed they wanted nominal load conditions, not worst case. Back to the drawing board. Upon resuming this effort, I found myself calculating resistances of number 36 AWG wire sizes having lengths of less than a half inch in some cases. Also, it was necessary to compute inductive as well as capacitive impedance, which in normal circumstances were so minute as to be negligible. Other than this, I had no idea what I was accomplishing, even when I was working with calibration loads for I.R. sensors. This project was the dullest, most lackluster effort for me of anything I was ever associated with at Hughes Aircraft Company.

On one occasion, I was assigned to the Environmental and Check-out Lab for this particular spy-in-the-sky, when two wires about 2 ½ inches long were found to have no support between their end connections. Two days were required for not less than eight different engineering groups to decide how to secure these wires to the chassis with a given type epoxy.

Then, when the job was undertaken, thirteen engineers were present in the lab to witness the operation, all of whom had to sign off on the effort. A total of four days were consumed to resolve this problem. I understood the reasoning for this process, yet it did not appeal to me from the standpoint of holding my interest. All environmental, as well as functional tests were most laborious and time consuming. On top of all this, we were in a "Clean Room Lab" where it was necessary to wear special dust free attire. Considering the product we were constructing and its mission in space, coupled with the necessity for it to operate flawlessly with no possibility for service or repair, this project was a challenge of the highest order.

Recognizing in myself no desire to pursue projects of this nature, I visited a section of Radar Systems Group that was engaged with providing a new state-of-the-art electronic weapons control system for one of our military aircraft. When I left, I had a new job starting the following week, based upon my performance in the F-14 program. However, on my way back to my office it occurred to me that I was 62 years old, and asked myself, why should I bust my ass to come upon the learning curve of a new system that would require many hours of overtime and much hard work to meet schedules. Why not retire?

As soon as I got to my office my mind was made up. I told my present supervisor of my intentions and called the person who would have been my new boss and informed him that I was retiring. Normally, the Personnel Department took 45 to 60 days to process a retirement. However, I talked real nice to a young lady there and she wrapped mine up in 30 days. Two hundred-fifty people attended my retirement luncheon. I retired from Hughes Aircraft Company on the last working day of the month, June 30, 1984 with the title of Development Engineer Specialist.

After 21 years in the U.S. Navy this day culminated another 25 years in Electrical Engineering. For most part, there were no two days alike during my career. New challenges occurred almost daily.

31

Second Retirement

All at once, I did not have to roll out of the hay at the crack of dawn and get ready to hit the freeway. Still, I found myself out of bed at 6:00a.m. having my first cup of coffee and planning what I was going to accomplish that day. One of my first undertakings was to build an extension onto my wooden stepladder. First, it was necessary to overhaul the old six-footer. Then I would extend it in height by 2 feet, thus giving it a height of eight-feet. It worked out beautifully and it is now a very sturdy ladder. It comes in mighty handy around the motor home as well as the house.

Other projects included rebuilding the old basket weave redwood fence along the north side of my property, in addition to replacing a number of fence posts. I completed half of the fence, but the half alongside the house was left leaning and tied against the high school chain-link fence. The reason being that Jaretta, who was in bad health to begin with was getting worse. My desire was to spend as much time with her as possible and take her wherever she wanted to go. She was my life.

One of my projects found Jaretta and me in an upholstery shop where we purchased foam padding and material for covering the seats of our dining chairs. They looked quite nice afterward, but I had some fingers that were quite sore on the tips.

About this time, we got the urge to take a vacation and visit our grandkids and relatives back in Texas, Oklahoma, and the mid-west.

First, however, it seemed proper to buy a new car. We visited our local Oldsmobile dealer and came away with a new 1986 Olds 98 four-door sedan, the color of desert sand. It was a real pleasure to drive this vehicle.

The first night we spent in Tucson, AZ, the second night in Pecas, TX and we arrived in Lewisville, TX on the third day. Upon arriving in Lewisville, I discovered I had left our granddaughter, Jodee's address and phone number at home. Finally, we got hold of number two granddaughter, Amber and her husband DeWayne. They managed to get us in touch with Jodee and her husband, Gary. Please be informed however, before we made contact with any of them I was so exasperated I was ready to move on without seeing any of them. As it turned out, we spent 4 days visiting Jodee and Gary. Amber and Dewayne, who lived about 30 miles away, came up on the weekend.

Next, we drove to Tulsa where we visited with my two sisters, Dorothy and Patty Jo and their families, both of whom lived in southwest Tulsa. I believe we stayed with Patty and Pat about 4 days, while during the day we would go over to Dorothy's which, was about a mile away. Upon departing from Dorothy and Patty's area, we drove up to Chuck's place (my brother) in Oswego, about 20 miles north of downtown Tulsa where we visited for about 3 days. During this time, my sister Charlotte Ann came to visit on the weekend.

32

Jaretta's Losing Battle

After leaving the Tulsa area, we went to Iowa where we spent 5 or 6 days with Jaretta's sister, Freda Hildebrand, and her family on the farm near Lamoni. Freda's husband, Ferd, and I managed to get in a little cat fishing while we were there. We then drove up to Frankfort, Michigan where her sister Clara Lancing and her husband, Bob lived. Freda and Ferd also drove up there from Iowa and brothers Anthony Jordan and his wife Juanita from Mt. Clemens, MI and Clarence from Ozark, Arkansas also gathered. It proved to be quite a family reunion. During our stay here we fished Lake Michigan for salmon and caught our fair share. On average, we would bring in 4 or 5 King Salmon weighing from 17 to 25 pounds. These Bob would dress out, cutting the filets into pieces small enough to fit into wide mouth pint jars. Clara would then, after soaking over night in a salt brine, can the fish in her pressure cooker. There was no fat, bone, nor skin canned with this fish. Suffice it to say there was plenty of fish for all to take some home upon leaving. This was quite a trip. I believe we were gone about 5 weeks.

While she seldom complained, I noticed from time to time Jaretta experienced a sharp pain in her chest. She was under the care of a group of doctors specializing in arthritis. First she was diagnosed as having both Osteo and Rheumatoid arthritis. Then after about a year of treatment for the foregoing, she was diagnosed as having Lupus. All this was prior to our trip back to Texas, Oklahoma, Iowa, and Michigan. We had been back home about 6 months when she began to experience breathing problems. The arthritis group of doctors recommended a group of Pulmonary Specialists. Jaretta was under the care of both groups of doctors for the rest of her life. At the time however, she seemed to be holding her own. On a visit to the pulmonary group, the latter part of January 1987, a dark spot about the size of a half dollar showed up in an X-ray of her lungs. This spot was closely watched for a couple weeks, and then a needle biopsy was taken the first part of March. Unfortunately, the resulting lab report disclosed Adeno-Carcenoma, a very mean cancer.

The doctors determined she could not take chemotherapy, which left radiation only. Upon her first scheduled radiation treatment, an X-ray of her lungs revealed so little healthy tissue left that radiation would have killed her outright. Should I live to be a thousand years old, I will never forget the expression of utter despair on Jaretta's face when informed of this situation. What made it worse for me was the fact there was absolutely nothing neither anyone nor I could do to comfort her.

Already Jaretta was beginning to experience considerable pain. A special prescription was prepared for liquid morphine, which she could take by mouth, but had to be filled at the hospital pharmacy only. I asked for a prognosis about the first of April and the doctor stated four months. She lasted two months. Those two months were the longest of my life.

33

Different Life

One of the most difficult tasks of my life was making arrangements for Jaretta's demise two months before she passed away. I do not believe I could have accomplished this without the presence of my eldest grandson, Ron. Upon learning of Jaretta's terminal condition, several of her brothers and sisters came to California for a final visit of a week or ten days. During this period, Jaretta was not yet confined to bed.

Following their departure, the situation became extremely difficult for Shirley, my daughter and I. The two of us nursed and tended Jaretta for nearly two months, to the very end. We each got very little sleep. It was almost impossible to keep her in bed. When I would manage to get a little sleep, I would awaken after a few minutes to find her standing at the foot of my bed. Nothing would do but to get up and put her back to bed then sit alongside her bed for hours. A quilt made by Jaretta's mother many years before was on her bed. One morning she was sitting in the middle of the bed identifying each piece of material in that quilt as to which of the girls her mother had made a dress.

Jaretta suffered a stroke of some sort that left her mouth drooped such that she could not take food nor medicine by mouth. It became necessary to take her to the hospital the morning of 27 May 1987. She passed away about 9:30 p.m. the night of 29 May 1987.

Following Jaretta's passing away, about six weeks after, I pulled myself together and set out on the longest trip of my life. First I went to Iowa to visit her eldest sister, Freda, and her husband Ferd Hildebrand.

After 4 or 5 days, I proceeded to Tomahawk, Wisconsin where I spent 3 or 4 days with Bob and Fran Leassig, old friends whom we had known for many years. From there, I drove across upper Michigan, crossed the Mackinac Straits Bridge then down to Bear Lake, Michigan to visit Jaretta's sister Clara and her husband Bob Lancing. While there her brother Tony and his wife Juanita came up to Bear Lake from Mt. Clemens. They stayed for about 5 days. We had a very nice visit, but I was always aware of a big void in my life. I left a couple days after Tony and Juanita departed. My next trip took me to Ozark, Arkansas, where I visited Jaretta's brother, Clarence Jordan. Spent a couple days there then journeyed to Lewisville, Texas, where our eldest granddaughter, Jodee and her husband Gary lived. After about 5 days there, I moved on, this time going to Tulsa, Oklahoma to see my sisters Dorothy, Patty, and Charlotte Ann and my brother Charles.

Before I started this trip, it was agreed I was to meet Al and Millie Herriford in Amarillo, Texas at Millie's stepfather's home. Al is my youngest uncle, my dad's youngest brother, although I am older than he is by 2 months, 3 weeks and 2 days. The idea was that from Amarillo we would caravan to Albuquerque, NM for the reunion of the USS Detroit, the light cruiser Al and I were aboard during the Pearl Harbor Attack. Period of the reunion was from Thursday 10th through Sunday 13th of September, 1987.

Unknown to me, Al and Millie had arranged for Doris Bassett, widow of Bob, a USS Detroit shipmate during the Pearl Harbor Attack, to fly to Albuquerque with the proviso that she would return to California by car. I was introduced to Doris almost immediately. She possessed a wonderful outgoing personality and we hit it off right away. However, we both had something in common that seemed to pull us together, that being we each had recently lost our spouses. Doris's husband, Bob Bassett passed away on 19 January, 1987 and Jaretta passed away on 29 May 1987. While we usually had a good time in company with friends, quite often for one reason or another one or sometimes both of us would find ourselves quietly shedding a few tears. Frankly, it was comforting to have one another to lean on.

Upon leaving Albuquerque, we decided to follow Don and Pauline Hollandsworth to their home in Casper, Wyoming. Doris rode with me as we followed the other two cars. On the way we spent a day at Royal Gorge and arrived in Casper the second day where we stayed a couple days. During over night stops in motels Doris and Millie shared one room while Al and I shared another. This arrangement held while at the Hollingsworth's also. From Casper we returned to California where I dropped Doris off at her home in Burbank. Following this Doris and I started seeing one another on a regular basis.

Al and Millie had me spend a weekend or two with them out in San Fernando Valley in Arleta. This was only about 8 miles from where Doris lived. I therefore took her out to dinner on a couple occasions. Al also was a member of Chapter 12, Pearl Harbor Survivors Association, (PHSA) that meets at the VFW hall in Burbank. Surviving spouses of deceased PHSA members are known as "Sweethearts" of which Doris was one. Both Al and I are life members of PHSA, but at this time, I was a member of National Chapter 1, located in Gardena. Al had just been elected President of Chapter 12 and among others persuaded me to transfer. This I did but refrained from submitting my papers until after the new slate of officers for Chapter 12 had been sworn into office.

The weekend following Chapter 12 installation of officers the Vice President and his wife were involved in an auto accident which took her life and placed him in the hospital for approximately 6 months. Now at the very next meeting of Chapter 12 guess who was appointed the new Vice President. Do you suppose this uncle of mine could be accused of "nepotism"? Seriously, however, I am thankful for this appointment. At this particular time in my life, I needed something into which I could become very deeply involved.

The Pearl Harbor Survivors Association proved to be the vehicle I needed to occupy my time and energy. Subsequently I have served as president and secretary of Chapter 12 and have gone on to become California Vice State Chairman, South 1990-1992; California State Chairman 1992-1994; Trustee on the California PHSA Executive Board 1994 to 1998 and am currently serving a second term as Vice State Chairman, South 1998-2000. At this time I am a candidate for the National office of First District Director in the election to be conducted at our PHSA State Convention in Redding in May 2000. During the period 1994 to 1998 I served as a Trustee on the California PHSA Executive Board. All past State Chairmen are supposed to serve in this capacity for a total of 6 years.

Soon after Doris and I started going together, I purchased a used motor home, which afforded us the ability to travel throughout the state to participate in various PHSA events. Doris and I traveled up and down the state with this rig for about 18 months. Later we traded it in for a new 1992 Bounder. Al and Millie also bought a new Southwind motor home about the same time. Together with many others who had motor homes, we traveled all up and down the state and across the U.S. as well as Canada and Mexico.

These days were wonderful. Some of our trips lasted for as long as 8 weeks at a time.

34

Doris

Doris and I traveled all over California and I believe I have become acquainted with nearly every Pearl Harbor Survivor in the state as well as many in Arizona and Nevada.

Doris was a very delightful person to be around. I do not believe she had an enemy in the world. Her daughter, Diane Anderson and husband Jim, whom we visited frequently, lived in Monrovia, about 25 miles from Doris's home in Burbank, California.

Doris worked as an escrow officer in a bank in Hollywood, CA while raising Diane and a son Randy. She divorced their father, Jim Sublett when the children were in their teens and Randy subsequently went to live with his father. However, the most remarkable thing about Doris was, as a single woman raising two teenage children she managed to obtain a loan with which to purchase a home. In the latter 1960's it was all, but impossible for a single woman to obtain such a loan. Let me tell you she was mighty proud of her home and in my opinion had every right to be.

Together, we went on six different cruises ranging from 4 to 16 days. We went to Alaska; the Caribbean; the New England coast, Nova Scotia and St. Lawrence River; from Puerto Rico through the Panama Canal to Los Angeles; and two different cruises from Florida to the Bahamas. On two occasions, we flew to Miami, Florida to visit Russell and Irma Richardson who lived down on the Keys. Irma was Bob Bassett's sister, Bob being Doris's late husband. Another time Doris and I along with Al and Millie Herriford visited the Richardson's, having driven down to the Keys in our motor homes.

We, in our motor homes, had made a trip to Norfolk, Virginia for a reunion of the USS Detroit. Al Herriford, Bob Bassett, and I were all three shipmates aboard the Detroit during the Pearl Harbor Attack on 7 December 1941. Doris and Irma were very close; therefore, we decided to make the trip from Norfolk down to the Keys being that we were already on the East Coast.

This proved to be quite a memorable trip. We encountered "Love-Bugs" in Georgia and Orlando, Florida. After 3 days of visiting Disney World, Epcot Center and Silver Springs Aquacades, our journey took us to Russ and Irma's on Plantation Key, Florida. Russ and Irma drove us down to Key West, a distance of about 96 miles from their home on Plantation Key.

The seafood experienced in various restaurants was delightful. Suffice it to say we enjoyed four wonderful days of Russ and Irma's hospitality. We departed about 5 O'clock in the morning, our destination being Tallahassee where we arrived about 8:00 PM, with the front of our motor homes covered with "Love-Bugs" again.

We stayed over night in the RV facility at the Elks lodge where we were treated like royalty. The following morning Al and I spent about 2-hours washing the front of our motor homes in order to remove "Love-Bugs". Later we came across a product for sale guaranteed to remove "Road-tar and Love-Bugs".

From Tallahassee, we followed highway I-10 west to New Orleans where we enjoyed a couple days of outstanding cuisine. Then to Houston, San Antonio, El Paso and on home to California, stopping only to spend the night. This trip spanned eight weeks.

Another time, Shirley and Gilbert Olinger, towing a 26-foot trailer, along with Al and Millie and Doris and I, started a trip to Canada. We crossed the Mojave Desert in 114 degree heat while temperatures of 95 to 105 degrees followed us all the way to Salt Lake City. On our way to Twin Falls, Idaho, we took a detour to Promontory, Utah where we participated in a reenactment of driving the golden spike at the joining of the transcontinental railroad. At Twin Falls, Gil took sick and had to be admitted to a hospital. Al and I relocated their trailer to an RV facility at the hospital so Shirley would have a place to stay, then Al and Millie, and Doris and I continued the trip to Canada in our motor homes. Our trip took us up through Banff to Jasper. From there, we looped back to the southwest through Kamloops, BC then to Vancouver. We took our motor homes on the ferry to Vancouver Island where we spent three days touring the Island and Victoria, after which, we took the ferry to Port Angeles, Washington. Subsequently, we visited Mt. Saint Helens then wound our way to Coos Bay, Oregon for the USS Detroit reunion where we again met Shirley and Gilbert.

Doris and I often visited Gilbert and Shirley Olinger in Van Nuys, also any time we passed through Selma when they were in residence there. Very often, they caravanned to various PHSA functions with us. Many is the time when we were in Selma, Gil and I would pick oranges, grapefruit, grapes, and steal Fuji Apples from his neighbor to bring back home. Usually there was so much, we gave most away when we returned home.

Gil had a knee replaced and while in the hospital his kidneys failed. He was in the hospital well over a month and upon release, required dialysis twice and sometimes three times a week. They purchased a class "C" motor home and we continued to travel. I could see Gil was becoming gradually worse. Then one day there was a call on my answering machine from Shirley. When I returned the call, Shirley informed me Gil had passed away the night before. They were in Selma at the time.

Shirley asked Bill Davis and me to officiate Gil's funeral. This we readily agreed to. However, the night before the funeral, Bill had an attack of hypoglycemia and had to be hospitalized. I therefore conducted the funeral alone, and was happy to do so for Shirley's sake.

After Shirley's first husband, Allen passed away Doris and I made a point of taking Shirley with us in the motor home to various functions. We both thought the world of her. Again, after Gil Passed away we took Shirley with us on several occasions. She was great company and we both enjoyed her very much.

Commencing in 1997, Doris was beginning to have much pain in her hips. She had arthroscopic surgery on one knee early in 1996 and was planning to have the other one done. Sometimes she hurt so bad just walking about the house, she would simply sit down and cry. Then one morning, using the walker we had borrowed from Joe and Thelma Mariani, she hurt so bad she had to rest after taking 6 or 8 steps. It scared the hell out of me. I rushed her to the doctor and it was all she could do to get up to his office. The diagnosis was congestive heart failure and pneumonia. Arrangements were made to put her in the hospital, but she could not be admitted until after 4:00pm. This was on 5 January and half of the hospital staff was out with flu. While it was necessary to return her home, I made sure she got admitted at 4:00pm. After the diagnosis in the doctors office Doris turned to me and asked, "Am I going to die?" I responded, "No way!" Little did I know at that time she would pass away eleven days later, on the night of 16th of January 1998.

I loved Doris very, very much. Her death was a terrible shock. During 10 1/2 years of our relationship, there was never a single cross word between us. She was always eager to go, regardless of how she might feel. We enjoyed each other's company to the fullest.

Shirley Olinger lost her husband, Gilbert in March of 1996. She, Doris and I had been very close friends for many years and it just seemed natural for the two of us to be drawn together. I was committed to attend the Gridley Clam Bake the latter part of April, 1998, but could not bear the thought of making that long drive, approximately 500 miles, alone. Therefore, I asked Shirley to accompany me. Actually, I had started seeing Shirley a few weeks earlier. We have been going together ever since. Under the circumstance, we have been very good for one another and have developed a love for one another that sustains us. I feel Doris would be the first to approve our relationship.

Together we are both involved with the Pearl Harbor Survivors Association and the Dick Salter Chapter for City of Hope fund raising. Both these organizations keep us quite busy, and still leave us time to travel.

This finds me in the twilight of life on 18 March 2000. I live each day as if it is the last, mind the doctors and Shirley and stay busy. At present my home is in Anaheim, while Shirley lives in Van Nuys, about 47 miles apart. We spend about equal time at each location. I consider myself extremely fortunate in that Shirley was there for me. Both of us were in need of companionship. This we have found in one another and in the process, a strong love has developed.

35

The Twilight Years

Several months following Doris's death Shirley and I commenced keeping company. We had known each other for many years. I am certain Doris would approve Shirley and me going together. Following our trip to Gridley for the 1998 Clam Bake, we went together for approximately two years, after which, we moved in together.

As a surprise to both of us, very often we found ourselves thinking the same thoughts even though only one of us would utter a single word. It's as if we were connected by a line of telepathy. In several other ways, these attributes become apparent from time to time. We became more and more conscious of our idiosyncrasies until we found ourselves deeply in love with one another. Although we are living together, we have a mutual understanding that at our age and for several good reasons, marriage is not in the picture because of financial impediments. I sold my home in Anaheim with the sale closing on 9 April 2001, and moved in with Shirley in Van Nuys.

It was a year earlier that I entered the hospital on 11 April 2000 with angina and was almost immediately admitted to the ICU. On the 14th of April I underwent a 4-way heart bypass operation. Two days following the heart operation blood tests revealed my Hemoglobin was down to 9. It should have been 14. This indicated I had lost 40% of my blood. My stools were absolutely black. I was taken into a lab where a scope was inserted down my throat into my stomach. Two bleeding ulcers were found and cauterized. These ulcers were brought on by a bacterial infection discovered in my stomach and lower intestines. I was put on a very heavy antibiotic over a period of three weeks, which left a very bitter taste in the mouth. At one time I counted eleven different bags of I.V. being administered to me. There were four different I.V. stops connected to me at one time, two in the back of the right hand, one in the back of the left hand and one in my neck. During the next couple days I received two whole blood transfusions, and was discharged from the hospital on 21 April 2000.

On 29 April I discovered a rash on my back just to the right of my spine and about an inch below my belt line. This was the beginning of "Shingles". Following is a write-up I performed relative to this malady:

CHRONOLOGY OF A TRIP TO HELL AND BACK

11 April 2000—I awoke about 5:00a.m. with a tightness in my chest and some angina pain. I got out of bed, went onto the kitchen, sat down at the table and placed a nitro pill under my tongue. After 5 minutes I still had the pain, so I took a second nitro pill. The pain let up so I went back to bed. About 6:00a.m. I again awoke with symptoms described above. Again I got up and sat at the kitchen table and proceeded with the same nitro procedure as before. After about 15 minutes, I felt all right.

Shirley had a doctor's appointment in Garden Grove, so we were preparing to drive down there. After loading light luggage into the car, the angina returned with tightness in my chest. I sat in a chair in the living room and again repeated the nitro pills procedure, whereupon the angina diminished. Shirley was not happy with my condition and she called my cardiologist in Garden Grove who recommended driving to Garden Grove Hospital Emergency. Shirley did not feel I could make the one hour drive to Garden Grove. She therefore drove me to Valley Presbyterian Hospital Emergency, a five minute drive from her house in Van Nuys. They took me in immediately after Shirley mentioned my heart condition. After all the various procedures were completed, the ER doctor informed me that I had earned at least a one night stay in their ICU. After being stabilized for a couple days the cardiologist determined I should be given an angiogram.

13 April 2000—The cardiologist presented me with the results of the angiogram that showed four partially blocked arteries. Later that afternoon the head surgeon of a heart surgery team from Cedar's Sinai Hospital convinced me I needed open heart surgery. This I agreed to and it was scheduled for 7:30 next morning.

14 April 2000—I was transported to the operating room at 7:30 a.m. The operation commenced about 8:30 and was completed about 12:30 p.m. when I was returned to ICU. From shortly before 8:30 the day was a complete blank to me.

15 April 2000—The head surgeon, Dr. Kass of the open heart surgical team, cut the stitches holding two black tubes inserted in my chest and pulled them out. That was the first thing I remember following the surgery. Sometime later, Dr Cheng, partner of Dr. Kass removed the respirator from my throat. I thought I was going to die when the tubes were partially pulled from my throat and left there for some period of time. I could not talk nor breathe and was literally chocking while waving my arms at the nurse. Finally the tubes were completely removed from my throat and it was a great relief to be breathing on my own.

16 April 2000—I was removed from the ICU and installed in a room that was monitored. Blood tests revealed I had a loss of blood. My hemoglobin was down to 9 and it should have been 14. This indicated a 40% loss of blood. My stools were absolutely Black.

18 April 2000—I was taken to a lab where an EGD was performed, (scope was inserted down my throat into my stomach). Two bleeding ulcers were discovered and cauterized. It was also found that I had a

bacterial infection in my stomach and lower intestines. This resulted in a course of heavy antibiotics which lasted for three weeks and caused a very bitter taste in my throat during some period of time after the medication had been taken. I was given a whole blood transfusion on this date.

20 April 2000—I received another whole blood transfusion today.

21 April 2000—I was released from the hospital to go home and recuperate.

29 April 2000—Discovered a rash on my back about an inch below the belt line and to the right of my spine, which we thought might be an allergic reaction to some of the medication I was taking. Up until now, everything was proceeding very well with my recuperation.

1 May 2000—I had an appointment with Dr. Chetty, the gastroenterologist. When Dr Chetty saw the rash, he was of the opinion that it was shingles and not an allergic reaction to medication. Not feeling too well, we called Dr. Pandian, the cardiologist and he had us come right over to see him. He checked me out and said all was well, but he too concurred with Dr. Chetty that the rash looked like shingles. He then arranged an emergency appointment with a dermatologist, Dr. Hartman. Dr. Hartman confirmed that the rash was indeed shingles. He gave me a shot of hydrocortisone in the right cheek of my butt and a weed's supply of Acyclovir, and antiviral medication, to be taken around the clock every four hours.

2 May 2000—By now I was experiencing excruciating pain continuously day and night without let-up. I could not eat or sleep and felt I was always on the verge of vomiting. I paced the floor day and night. Several times I had the thought that if I could get my hands on a gun I would end it all, I hurt so badly. Pain from the heart surgery was negligible. The pain consisted primarily from the shingles and severe spinal arthritis. The combined pain was absolutely hell.

5 June 2000—After 5 weeks of pure hell, the pain level diminished to approximately 60% of worse case condition. This is due to a new medication, Neurontin, prescribed by Dr Hartman.

16 June 2000—I was given a treadmill at the hospital to determine at what level to start Cardio rehab.

21 June 2000—The pain level is down to about 40% of peak.

23 June 2000—Dr. Chetty performed another EGD to see how well the ulcers were doing. All was O.K.

27 June 2000—One Shingles ulcer about the size of a nickel remains on right side of spine and pain level is about 30% of peak. All other lesions are healing well, but the exposed nerve pain continues.

3 July 2000—Pain level still remains about 30% of peak. At the present rate of recovery, it will be August 1st or later before I am over this. On 17 August 2000, I still had the tail end of Shingles and indications are that it will hang on until about the end of the year. I have since learned that Shingles never completely disappear.

It has taken me a full year to recover from the year of ill health therefore comprising almost two year's total. Commencing 1 January 2002 I began feeling like a human being again. Shirley has nurtured my recovery all the way. There is absolutely no way I can express my love and gratitude for this wonderful lady that is justifiable. I thank almighty God I have her to lean on.

Note: Had it not been for Shirley's tender loving care, I would not have survived this ordeal. She is an angel in disguise, and I love her dearly.

Art Herriford

0-595-34242-6

www.ingramcontent.com/pod-product-compliance
Lightning Source LLC
Chambersburg PA
CBHW020426290526
45784CB00012BA/313